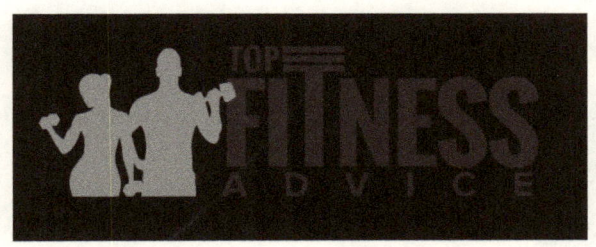

DETOX

3rd Edition

3-Day Weight Loss Detox Diet & Body Cleanse (With Detox Juice & Smoothie Recipes And Meal Plan)

LINDA WESTWOOD

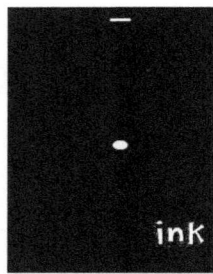

First published in 2015 by Venture Ink Publishing

Copyright © Top Fitness Advice 2019

All rights reserved.

No part of this book may be reproduced in any form without permission in writing from the author. No part of this publication may be reproduced or transmitted in any form or by any means, mechanic, electronic, photocopying, recording, by any storage or retrieval system, or transmitted by email without the permission in writing from the author and publisher.

Requests to the publisher for permission should be addressed to publishing@ventureink.co

For more information about the contents of this book or questions to the author, please contact Linda Westwood at linda@topfitnessadvice.com

Disclaimer

This book provides wellness management information in an informative and educational manner only, with information that is general in nature and that is not specific to you, the reader. The contents of this book are intended to assist you and other readers in your personal wellness efforts. Consult your physician regarding the applicability of any information provided in this book to you.

Nothing in this book should be construed as personal advice or diagnosis, and must not be used in this manner. The information provided about conditions is general in nature. This information does not cover all possible uses, actions, precautions, side-effects, or interactions of medicines, or medical procedures. The information in this book should not be considered as complete and does not cover all diseases, ailments, physical conditions, or their treatment.

You should consult with your physician before beginning any exercise, weight loss, or health care program. This book should not be used in place of a call or visit to a competent health-care professional. You should consult a health care professional before adopting any of the suggestions in this book or before drawing inferences from it.

Any decision regarding treatment and medication for your condition should be made with the advice and consultation of a qualified health care professional. If you have, or suspect you have, a health-care problem, then you should immediately contact a qualified health care professional for treatment.

No Warranties: The author and publisher don't guarantee or warrant the quality, accuracy, completeness, timeliness, appropriateness or suitability of the information in this book, or of any product or services referenced in this book.

The information in this book is provided on an "as is" basis and the author and publisher make no representations or warranties of any kind with respect to this information. This book may contain inaccuracies, typographical errors, or other errors.

Liability Disclaimer: The publisher, author, and other parties involved in the creation, production, provision of information, or delivery of this book specifically disclaim any responsibility, and shall not be held liable for any damages, claims, injuries, losses, liabilities, costs, or obligations including any direct, indirect, special, incidental, or consequences damages (collectively known as "Damages") whatsoever and howsoever caused, arising out of, or in connection with the use or misuse of the site and the information contained within it, whether such Damages arise in contract, tort, negligence, equity, statute law, or by way of other legal theory.

Table of Contents

Disclaimer	3
Who is this book for?	7
What will this book teach you?	9
Introduction	11
Chapter One: Why It Works	15
Chapter Two: Prepare Before the Weekend	21
Chapter Three: Starting the Detox	45
Chapter Four: What You're Drinking	57
Breakfast Drinks	63
Lunch Drinks	75
Dinner Drinks	87
Chapter Five: Lose Up To 10 Pounds!	103
Chapter Six: Be Safe	109
Chapter Seven: Next Weekend	115
Chapter Eight: Do It Again	135
Conclusion	139
Final Words	141

Would you prefer to listen to my book, rather than read it?

Download the audiobook version for free!

If you go to the special link below and sign up to Audible as a new customer, you can get the audiobook version of my book completely free.

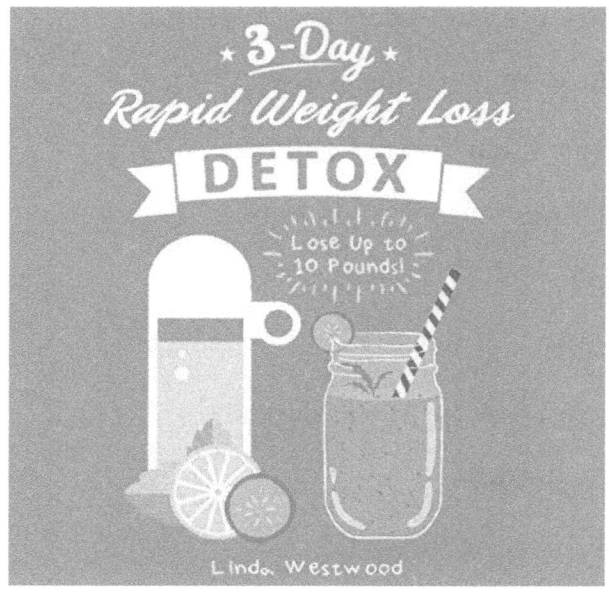

Go here to get your audiobook version for free:

TopFitnessAdvice.com/go/detox

Who is this book for?

Do you need a *strong* kick-start with your weight loss?

Do you need to lost weight *FAST*?

Do you have an event coming up that you need to *shed pounds fast* for?

If you answered "Yes" to any of those questions – **this book is for you!**

I am going to share with you the most effective way to rapidly lose weight and detox your mind and body in just 3 days!

I have put it all together in this awesome Weekend Weight Loss plan!

The best part about is that you are going to see amazing results and this will *TRANSFORM YOUR BODY (inside and outside) IN JUST 3 DAYS*!

You can be a complete beginner or someone who works out regularly, it doesn't matter!

If this sounds like it could help you, then keep reading…

What will this book teach you?

Inside, I will teach you one of the best ways to quickly lose weight, especially targeted to cleansing your body with a 3-day detox!

You will feel the healthiest you have ever felt – have the most energy you have ever had – and the fat will be melting *constantly!*

How? Because you're going to be consuming the right things to cleanse your body in a short period of time.

In this book, I give you the plan right in front of you that will change your life – all you have to do is follow it!

One of the most important things for you to realize when reading this book is that this weight loss plan *really does work!*

However…

For you to achieve *real success*, you HAVE to apply this to your life.

This is where most people fail – they read through the entire book but do nothing.

You MUST try your best to apply as you read through the book!

Introduction

Are you struggling to lose weight? You are not alone. 30 percent of the world's population is overweight or obese.

Why does it matter? What makes millions of people endeavor to lose weight each year?

Frankly, health. Obesity can lead to high blood pressure, diabetes, osteoarthritis, heart disease and coronary artery disease, fatty liver, sleep apnea, and certain kinds of cancer.

Many people who begin a weight loss regimen do not continue because even when they eat a healthy diet and exercise they cannot seem to lose weight.

However, if you are losing the battle of the bulge, the problem might not be your diet. It might be within your body itself.

Slow Metabolism

Metabolism refers to the efficiency with which your body burns calories for energy. The "speed" of your metabolism, whether it is fast or slow, coincides with the ease of losing weight.

Many factors can have an effect of the speed of your metabolism. Your fitness level and your body composition, that is the ratio of muscle to fat, will affect it. If you carry more muscle, you burn calories more quickly.

Your age has tremendous influence on your metabolism. When you are young, you have a speedy metabolism that burns off calories very quickly.

Do you look back longingly at your teenage years when you could eat anything and not gain weight?

You were able to eat like that because your metabolism was lightning fast. But, as you age your metabolism slows down.

Even in your 20s your metabolism can stay pretty fast and keep you slim. But after you turn 30 your metabolism slows down a lot and that can lead to weight gain.

Your metabolism will continue to slow down as you age. So, unless you find a solution that works for you, it will just get more and more difficult to lose weight.

It is, however, possible to speed it back up, and your detox is a good precursor to the healthy lifestyle that will do just that.

Body Pollution

Another factor that can make it hard to lose weight is years of body pollution.

All that fast food, refined sugar, and extra calories can take a huge toll on your body. Your liver, which is what processes wastes in the body, may not continue functioning effectively because it's been working overtime.

When you eat an unhealthy diet, fail to exercise and do not take care of yourself for years at a time, your body suffers. The effects of all those harmful years can make your body sluggish and polluted, which can make it tough to lose weight.

Detox and Weight Loss

If you want to kick start weight loss or cleanse your body so that it functions as effectively as possible, a detox is the way to go.

Detox is short for detoxification, and it is the process by which we remove toxins from our systems. Participating in a detox can be less than pleasant, but it will rejuvenate your body, clean out the pollution and toxins, and make it easier for you to lose weight.

Additionally, a liquid diet is effective for weight loss.

While the 3-day detox diet is designed only for use over a short time period, similar diets are used to lose tremendous amounts of weight, with a doctor's supervision.

There are many other weight loss programs that suggest two shakes a day and a "sensible" dinner. So, it should come as no surprise that the 3-day detox diet, being completely liquid, can perform amazingly to assist you in losing up to 10 pounds in one short weekend.

Chapter One

Why It Works

What happens to cars that never have an oil change? The buildup of sludge will destroy the motor. The same thing happens in your body when you do not take care of yourself.

If you stopped showering tomorrow what would happen to your skin?

Dirt would build up. Pollutants from the environment would build up. Your skin would look terrible, with probable breakouts, even rashes.

Your skin would also *feel* terrible. It would be itchy. Bacteria and toxins would build up and might cause sores and infections. So to prevent that you shower and wash with soap frequently.

Detox does the same thing for your internal systems that showering does for your skin. Over the years, all those pollutants and bacteria and other toxic chemicals in your body build up. They slow down your body's waste disposal system and make it difficult for your body to function.

You may gain weight, or have a harder time losing weight. Additionally, you may frequently feel exhausted, or lethargic. It may seem as if you are moving in a fog all the time. If your liver isn't filtering toxins out of your body the way it should you might find yourself getting sick more often.

An Internal Cleansing

When you go on a detox, you are giving your body a break from the daily barrage of fat, sugar, and other unhealthy pollutants to which you subject it. At the same time that you are giving your body a rest from breaking down and processing unhealthy foods, you are feeding it with healthy foods, such as fruits, vegetables and nuts.

Those healthy foods, when combined as the 3-day detox diet explains, will flush the toxins and bacteria out of your organs, your bloodstream, and everywhere else in your body. This will get your circulation and waste disposal systems working at full capacity again.

Once your body is running on all cylinders again it will be able to break down fat for energy and you will start to lose weight. It will also get rid of all the excess waste and nasty debris in your body that could be keeping you from losing weight and feeling your best.

Think of your body as being a living machine. All machines need maintenance. You don't expect your car to run forever with no maintenance, so why do you expect it of yourself? If you want your body to be a fat burning machine, sometimes you need to give it a little tune up so that it will work the way it is supposed to work. A detox is exactly the kind of maintenance that your body needs to begin metabolizing food more efficiently.

There are several additional benefits to your 3-day detox.

The 3-day detox diet may bolster your immune system. Once your waste disposal system is cleaned out, your focus on vitamin rich super foods should serve to supercharge your immune system.

The detox will improve the appearance and clarity of your skin. The epidermis, or skin, is the body's largest organ. Of course, the removal of toxins will reflect in your skin. Although you may experience patchy, itchy skin, or even an increase in breakouts at the beginning of the program, by the end of it you should see beautiful results.

The 3-day detox can help you regain your focus of mind. Some followers of the program say that detoxing cleared up fuzzy thinking and got their bodies and minds in balance.

Detoxing can give you healthier hair. Many people have said that removing the toxins from their bodies allowed their hair to grow faster and become healthier.

The 3-day detox can have anti-aging benefits. The buildup of toxins is one of the major causes of the effects we think of as aging. The process of clearing out impurities tackles free radicals that cause us to look and feel older.

As you can see, the 3-day detox can deliver much more in addition to weight loss!

Discover Scientifically-Proven "Shortcuts" & "Hacks" to Lose Weight FASTER (With Very Little Effort)

For this month only, you can get Linda's best-selling & most popular book absolutely free – *Weight Loss Secrets You NEED to Know*.

Get Your FREE Copy Here:

TopFitnessAdvice.com/Bonus

Discover scientifically-proven tips to help you lose weight faster and easier than ever before. With this book, readers were able to improve their weight loss results and fitness levels. So, it's highly recommended that you get this book, especially while it's free!

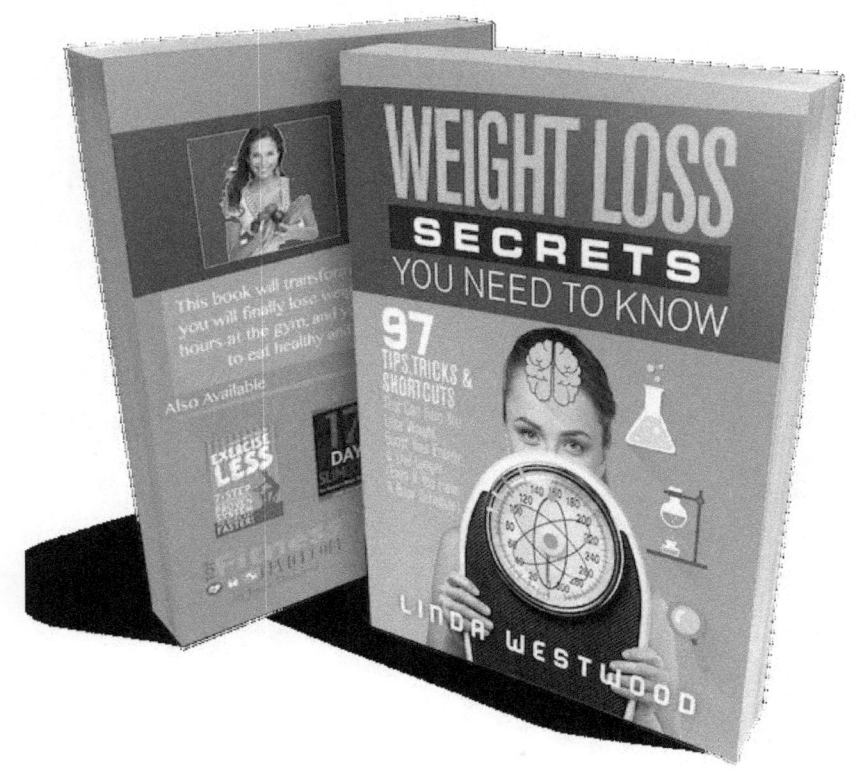

Get Your FREE Copy Here:

TopFitnessAdvice.com/Bonus

Chapter Two

Prepare Before the Weekend

The best way to do a 3-day detox is to pick a weekend that you can focus on yourself. You should plan on staying home for most of that weekend.

If you are doing the detox to lose weight before going to a wedding, a banquet, or another special occasion, it is a smart idea to do the detox a week in advance of the event. That will give you time to recover and look great at the event. Don't worry; you won't gain back the weight in a week.

Why Do It on A Weekend?

Doing the 3-day detox on a weekend is highly recommended. You probably should not attempt to drag yourself to work when you don't feel or look your best.

A detox is great for your body once it is done. However, you might feel cranky or even more sluggish and tired while you are actually engaged in the detox. This reaction is due to your body working overtime getting rid of so many toxins and other unhealthy pollutants from your system.

So, plan on taking a 3-day weekend to do the detox. You deserve it!

Make it at a spa weekend for yourself. Get some movies that you have been wanting to watch, load up on books and magazines, and plan on staying in your pajamas and pampering yourself all weekend.

By the time the detox is done you will be rested, and you will feel great. You will also be up to ten pounds lighter and your skin will be glowing. You will look fabulous for that special event.

Shop in Advance

Once you have picked a weekend to focus on your 3-day detox, you should take the time to create a shopping list. You will want to get all the items that you will need to do the detox in advance.

Going to the store during the detox will just tempt you to buy and eat a bunch of unhealthy food, and you will likely not feel up to it. One of the most important elements of any healthy lifestyle change is planning ahead. Another is avoiding temptation!

So, it is smarter to buy everything you are going to need ahead of time. That way you have no reason to go to the store and no excuse to go off of the detox diet. Making a complete shopping list ahead of time will also ensure that you have everything you need to do the detox.

Your health and the success of the 3-day detox depends upon following the plan, and you can only do that if you have all the ingredients.

Ordering Supplies

Shopping in advance will also make it easier to find the items that you need to do the detox properly. Of course, you will have no trouble finding things like fruit and vegetables at the grocery store.

However, you might have a hard time finding the supplements that you need, some of the additional ingredients for the detox drinks, and the essential oils that you need for a detox bath. Thinking and planning ahead ensures that you will know if you can buy what you need or if you'll have to order it.

If you discover that you live in an area where items like those listed above can be difficult to procure, you will probably have to order some of them online.

Start researching the best shopping sites for those items as soon as you pick the weekend that you want to do to the detox. Order immediately, so that they will arrive in time. Another benefit to this approach is that if you decide to do the detox again for another event you will already have those items on hand.

Buy Organic and Local

When you buy the fruits and vegetables that you will be eating on the detox make a special effort to buy organic or local vegetables and fruit.

You are doing this detox to make your body healthy, so do not start out by eating unhealthy GMO fruit and vegetables which may introduce more pollutants and toxins into your system.

Remember that you are what you eat. If you want to be healthy, you must eat healthy food. Treating yourself and spending a little bit of extra money for organic or local produce is worth it for this purpose.

Once your body has detoxed you should use the lessons you will learn and make an effort to eat higher quality foods. You know you should stay away from processed food, refined sugar, and high fructose corn syrup and the 3-day detox will get you started down that healthy path.

Organic food, especially locally grown organic food, is richer in nutrients than conventionally grown food. Organic food is not exposed to chemical pesticides and fertilizers, and so will not reintroduce the toxins you are trying to flush out with the 3-day detox.

Local foods in particular retain more vitamins and minerals simply because they fresher.

Where to Shop for Local and Organic Foods

If you have a local natural foods store or food co-op you should be able to find plenty of organic choices of fruit and vegetables there.

You may be able to find the supplements and other supplies that you need there as well. Many natural food stores and co-ops carry spices, supplements, teas, and even the essential oils that you will need for your relaxing detox baths.

Some communities have a program called Community Supported Agriculture, or farm sharing. If you belong to a farm share, you pay for a crate of locally grown organic vegetables and fruit and you pay the farmer directly.

Some require an upfront payment for a season, but some you can join anytime. You might want to check out local farms to see if they have the fruits and vegetables that you need and if they have a farm-sharing program.

If not, you can find local farmer's markets online and see what fruits and vegetables you can find there. It's best to look at the organic section even here, because some farmers include store bought produce to sell more variety.

If you cannot find any organic or local vegetables and fruits you can still do the detox, but using organic vegetables and fruits is the best choice.

Vitamins and Supplements

While you are on the detox, you will be drinking every meal and you will not eat any solid food. To ensure that you get your required nutrition, you need to take a very high-quality multivitamin supplement for the duration of the detox.

Many of the nutrients that your body requires to function will be coming from the multivitamin during the detox.

That is because the detox is going to be working on flushing all the nasty stuff out of your body. Taking a multivitamin will be giving your body the vitamins and minerals it needs to keep functioning while the detox gives your organs and cells a good flushing.

You Need a Multivitamin

As any nutritionist will tell you, you should really be taking a high-quality multivitamin supplement each day anyway. A good multivitamin can help your body stay healthy. It also will help you maintain a healthy weight.

Your body knows what it needs and it serves these needs with cravings. If you are getting the nutrition you need, you will find it easier to stick to any eating plan you have.

Even if you eat a very healthy diet there are going to be times when you don't get enough of certain vitamins and minerals. Some minerals can't be gotten from commonly available foods and have to be taken in supplement form. Some vitamins and minerals are there in the foods that you eat, but not in the sufficient quantities to help you stay healthy.

So, investing in a high-quality multivitamin is going to benefit you even after you are done with the detox, as you begin a healthier lifestyle. Don't stop taking it just because the detox is over.

How to Choose a High-Quality Multivitamin

Have you ever looked at the vitamin aisle at the local pharmacy or grocery store? There are hundreds of choices when it comes to multivitamins!

More so, if you go to a health food store or a specialty supplement store, there are even more choices. It can be extremely challenging to try to choose a good quality vitamin when there are so many on the market. According to their labels, every single one is the best! It can seem nearly impossible to choose.

However, there is one fool proof way to be sure that the vitamins you are buying is good quality. According to nutrition experts, if you want to buy a high-quality vitamin it does not matter which one you buy as long as the vitamins come from food.

Synthetic Vitamins vs. Food Based Vitamins

Wait a minute, all vitamins do not come directly from food?

That sounds crazy, doesn't it?

It seems counterintuitive, but it can be true. In order to make vitamins cheaper to produce some companies use synthetic vitamins that are created in a lab.

Other vitamin companies break down actual food and extract the vitamins from it. Vitamins from food ingredients have the highest quality nutrition to help you stay healthy. That is the kind you want to buy.

Why Synthetic Vitamins Are Bad for Your Body

The human body is a complex organism. When the body breaks down food in order to get the vitamins and minerals out, it does not isolate each individual vitamin.

It uses those vitamins in pairs or groups to make it easier for different parts of the body to use those vitamins.

Vitamin C Isn't Just Vitamin C

As an example, take a look at Vitamin C. You need Vitamin C to stay healthy. It boosts the immune system. It keeps your cells healthy. It has been linked to cancer and stroke prevention, and even eye health.

Some food scientists say that Vitamin C can even help you live longer. Perhaps most important during your 3-day detox, Vitamin C helps your body absorb and process all of the other vitamins and minerals in your detox drinks

The base of Vitamin C is Ascorbic Acid, but the Vitamin C that is in food is a lot more than just Ascorbic Acid. Research shows that Vitamin C should be considered a complex of C vitamins, in a similar way to the Vitamin B Complex that is available. It also has trace amounts of other vitamins and minerals, called phytonutrients, that all work together with Vitamin C to make your body stronger.

Vitamin C that comes from food will be more complex, and have those tiny quantities of other vitamins and minerals that you need, but synthetic vitamins will have only Ascorbic Acid.

Ascorbic acid alone does not have nearly the benefits for your body provided by a natural form of Vitamin C.

Synthetic Vitamins Are a Waste in More Ways Than One

Synthetic vitamin and mineral supplements are created in the lab, but even scientists claim that they are "essentially" the same as those from food.

However, they are not identical chemically, and hence the body may not even recognize them as nutrients. Some of these manufactured supplements may even be seen as *toxins by the body*.

Science is only now beginning to understand phytonutrients and how they contribute to our health.

How can science possibly duplicate something it does not even understand?

Additionally, since synthetic vitamins do not have those paired up vitamins and minerals, the body does not know how to process them effectively.

Most of the time the body will not even process synthetic vitamins and they just end up getting washed out of the body with other wastes. Taking synthetic vitamins is a lot like flushing money down the drain.

Pick a Plant Based Multivitamin

When you are detoxing your body will need the best supplemental vitamins and minerals you can give it. So, in order to give your body the support that it needs while you are on the 3-day detox look for a supplement that uses vitamins and minerals from food.

To find out if a vitamin is food based or synthetic check the back of the label carefully. Vitamins that are plant based will usually have a long list of vitamins that are in the multivitamin.

The label usually will say that the vitamins come from food.

If the label doesn't say where the vitamins come from a surefire way to tell is to look at the listing for Vitamin C. If the label says Vitamin C, then the supplement is plant based. If it is labeled Ascorbic Acid then you can be pretty confident that the vitamin is synthetic.

Organic Vitamins

If you are buying your supplements at a local natural foods store, you might wonder if a higher priced organic vitamin is worth the extra cost. Some foods are really not worth paying more for an organic label, but vitamins are worth paying more for.

The organic label on a multivitamin means that the ingredients in the supplement come from organic food, which is extremely beneficial to your health. A "raw" food label is a plus. Organic and raw foods have the highest levels of vitamins and minerals.

So if buying an organic vitamin is an option, you should spend more to get an organic or raw food multivitamin. Take this 3-day detox as an opportunity to not only lose weight but also start taking better care of your body.

Taking care of your body starts with investing in better quality food and supplements. When the detox is done, you will feel rejuvenated. Eating high quality organic food and taking a high-quality multivitamin will keep you feeling great after the detox is over, and it will help you maintain your weight loss.

The next thing that you will need to make your 3-day detox a success is a good probiotic.

What Is a Probiotic?

Probiotics are certain forms of bacteria that are essential to your health. We think of bacteria as harmful, but some we actually need for our systems to work properly.

The term "probiotics" was coined to differentiate between the two. If you don't have enough probiotics in your body, or if the harmful bacteria are out of balance with the helpful bacteria, you can develop a lot of uncomfortable and unhealthy conditions.

Probiotics work with your body to keep it functioning the way it should.

Why You Need a Probiotic

Did you know that your body has both good bacteria and bad bacteria?

Good bacteria keep your body balanced and help your body prevent illnesses. Good bacteria prevent things like diarrhea, gas, bloating, infection, and many other illnesses and conditions. Bad bacteria can also cause skin problems like eczema and rashes.

You always have good bacteria and bad bacteria in your gut. But when the balance of those bacteria is out of whack it can cause some pretty serious problems.

This is another area science is only beginning to understand. Lots of things can cause an imbalance of bacteria in your body like:

- Getting sick
- Eating an unhealthy diet
- Taking certain medicines like antibiotics
- Eating too much sugar
- Stress

Taking a probiotic will introduce good and helpful bacteria back into your body. Those bacteria can restore the balance that you need to have in your gut in order to be healthy.

When you are doing the 3-day detox taking a probiotic will help get rid of the overabundance of negative bacteria and waste products that you are going to be flushing out of your body.

You can get some probiotic benefits from eating yogurt, because yogurt contains a very powerful and helpful probiotic agent. But, since you will not be eating any solid food on the 3-day detox you will need a probiotic supplement to bring your body into balance.

How to Choose a Probiotic

Choosing a probiotic supplement can be even more confusing than choosing a multivitamin.

In order to find a high-quality probiotic, you might need to go to a health food store or even order one on-line. A multitude of factors affect your choice of a quality supplement.

Live and Active Cultures

Have you ever noticed on a yogurt label the phrase "live and active cultures"? That means that the bacteria in the yogurt are the kind that is good for you. The key thing you need to look for when choosing a probiotic is that the probiotic contains live and active cultures.

Probiotics are regulated as food, so there is no guarantee of quality. You must carefully read the labels to avoid buying a probiotic supplement that will not provide the healthy bacteria you need.

The probiotic supplement is required to give information on what it contains right on the label. Probiotics are made up of healthy bacteria, which are living organisms. So, the bacteria need to be alive when you take them in order for them to do any good.

Viable Through the End of Shelf Life

A high-quality probiotic will also say on the label that the bacteria are "Viable through the end of shelf life." If the label doesn't say that it means that the bacteria aren't guaranteed to be alive when you take them.

Avoid any probiotic that says, "Viable at the time of manufacture" on the label. That means that the company only guarantees that the bacteria were alive when the supplement left the factory.

More Tips for Choosing a Probiotic

If you are still having trouble finding a good probiotic, you can use these tips to find one that will get your body back in balance and make the 3-day detox even more effective:

- Look for one with at least 20 different strains of bacteria. The more strains of bacteria the better.

- Look for one with one encapsulated pills, or other delayed rupture technology. That will keep the bacteria alive until you take it, and protect it from your stomach acids so that it arrives intact to your intestines.

- Check out the storage requirements. Some probiotic supplements need to be refrigerated but others merely require a cool dark place. Any probiotic supplement should be kept away from heat moisture.

- CFUs, or colony forming organisms, are the measure of how many good bacteria are included in your supplement, and you should be looking for 5 billion or above.

- Look for certification by a third party. Probiotics are not regulated as medicines, but as food, so choose a brand certified for quality by an independent organization.

Omega 3 Fatty Acids

The last supplement that you need to do the 3-day detox is an Omega 3 supplement. You are probably already familiar with Omega 3 fatty acids and the benefits they have for the body.

There are three main types of Omega 3 fatty acids. These are EPA, which helps with inflammation, DHA, which is essential for your brain's healthy functioning, and ALA, which your body can convert to either of the others.

Usually Omega 3 fatty acids are found in fish and fish oil, but they are also found in nuts and flax seeds. Omega 3 supplements are usually concentrated fish oil that is put into capsules. Some people worry that these supplements can have an odiferous, fishy smell, but that usually only happens if they are low quality or old. Regardless, they have a number of healthy benefits for the body.

Lowering Triglycerides

Triglycerides are a type of unhealthy fat. When you consume excess calories, your body first converts them into triglycerides. When you have high triglyceride levels you are at a elevated risk of having a heart attack. Taking an Omega 3 supplement can lower the triglycerides in your blood and lower your risk of heart attack.

Other Benefits of Omega 3 Fatty Acids

In addition to lowering your risk of a deadly heart attack Omega 3 fatty acids also:

- Lower your risk of developing dementia
- Help your memory
- Protect brain function and eyesight
- Promote healthy skin and nails

Omega 3 Fatty Acids and the 3-day Detox

Taking an Omega 3 fatty acid supplement during the 3-day detox will keep your brain functioning the way it should. Usually carbs and protein keep you alert, focused, and functioning.

Since you are going to be flushing out your body with a completely liquid diet for 3-days these fish oil supplements will make sure that you are alert and focused instead of fatigued and sleepy.

Detox Baths

Another element of the 3-day detox program is to take a detoxifying bath each day. The detox bath is an important part of the program and you shouldn't skip it. In order to prepare the detox bath, you will need Epsom salts and Lavender essential oil.

What Epsom Salts Do

Most of the bath bombs and bath salts that are sold use Epsom salts as a base. Epsom salts are gentle on the skin but are great for detoxifying the skin.

Epsom salts gently exfoliate the skin and improve circulation. They pull all the toxins from the skin and body. Additionally, Epsom salts relieve bodily aches and pains, and this will be comforting to your body as it goes through the detox.

You may find that you like the relaxing detox bath and want to make it a regular part of your relaxation practice. Epsom salts are inexpensive and you can find them at any pharmacy.

You can mix them with different flowers, herbs, or oils to make your bath aromatic as well as therapeutic.

Lavender Essential Oil

For this bath to be effective you need to use a Lavender essential oil that is 100% essential oil and not fragrance oil. Essential oils are extracted from the leaves and flowers of plants. They have many benefits.

Aromatherapy uses pure essential oils to help people relax and to treat medical conditions. Lavender essential oil is one of the gentlest essential oils. It is even used on babies to help them sleep and relax.

Lavender smells wonderful.

Adding Lavender essential oil to your bath will help you relax, improve your quality of sleep, and heal your skin. Lavender oil is often used to treat skin conditions like dry skin, eczema, rashes, burns, and acne.

Adding this essential oil to your bath water will make your skin soft and beautiful after the Epsom salts have pulled all the gross pollutants, dead skin and other harmful elements out of your body.

Substitutions

If you don't like the scent of Lavender essential oil you can use another gentle essential oil. Tea Tree essential oil is a great choice, as it has many of the same positive benefits of Lavender.

Just make sure that whatever oil you use is a pure essential oil and not a fragrance oil. Fragrance oils are synthetic and made to be used in perfumes and soaps. They have no healing benefits.

Some detox baths include apple cider vinegar, sea salt, baking soda, or ginger. You may decide you would like to try including these. They cause you to sweat, which aids the Epsom salts in drawing toxins out of your body.

The 3-day Detox Shopping List

Remember to get organic fruits and vegetables whenever possible for the best nutrition. You may get more of each item if you want, in case you need it, but the amount given is the minimum suggested amount to buy.

The list might look overwhelming. However, you will be given a choice of several drinks for each meal.

The following list is composed as if you were going to make all of them. Of course, in 3 days, you will only sample a few. So, here is where planning ahead comes in very handy.

Look ahead to Chapter 4, and see which drinks sound best to you. It will be a snap to stick to your liquid diet if you enjoy the drinks!

After picking out your tasty liquid meals, narrow the master list to a shopping list for those detox drinks you decided on. Once you have refined your list, stick to it.

You will thereby have an easier time sticking to your plan of completing the 3-day detox. Make sure that you also have a blender or juicer at home to make the drinks you will be drinking in place of actual meals.

Shopping List

- 5 cups raspberries
- 6 cups blueberries
- 4 cups strawberries
- 3 cups cranberries
- 1 cup green grapes
- 5 mangos
- 3 pineapples
- 6 apples, 4 green, 2 red
- 8 bananas
- 4 pears
- 1 cup pitted cherries
- 2 oranges
- 10 lemons
- 10 limes
- 6 dates
- 10 cups of kale
- 5 cups romaine lettuce
- 2 cups red leafed lettuce
- 1 bunch broccoli
- 3 avocadoes
- 5 cucumbers
- 5 cup of spinach
- 18 stalks of celery
- 3 large tomatoes

- 2 red bell peppers
- 1 bundle of watercress
- 1 bundle cilantro
- 1 large root jicama
- 4 cloves of garlic
- 5 carrots
- 1 pint local honey, any variety
- 1 pint unsweetened cranberry juice
- 1 pint unsweetened pineapple juice
- 1 pint unsweetened lemon juice
- 2 liters of coconut water
- 3 cartons of almond milk
- 2 ounces (50 grams) of matcha green tea
- Cayenne pepper
- Ground flax seeds
- Whole flax seeds
- 1 fingers Turmeric
- Cinnamon
- Nutmeg
- Almond butter
- Coconut oil
- Green Tea
- Stevia natural sweetener
- 1 large ginger root
- Mint leaves

Bath ingredients

- 2.5 cups of Epsom salts per bath
- Lavender essential oil (or your chosen substitute)+

How to Get Through the 3-day Detox

Even though you will feel rejuvenated after you are done with the detox and you will have lost a large amount of weight, it can be difficult to get through.

It is no fun not to eat for 3-days and only drink health drinks. You can expect to feel tired, cranky, and a little sick at times. This is because the drinks and baths will be bringing all the toxins and sludge in your body to the surface and then flushing it away.

So, it is totally normal to not feel at your best while you are going through the detox. That is why it is nearly essential to lay low for the 3-days of the plan. Of course, if you are normally an active person that much down time combined with not feeling well can be hard to take.

Instead of seeing the 3-day detox as something that you have to survive, though, you should look at it as a chance to have a mini-vacation to renew your spirit as well as your body.

Here are some fun ways make the weekend more restful, more interesting, and more rejuvenating:

- Turn your home into a home spa. Make homemade facemasks and other spa treatments to make you feel and look better.
- Pay a stylist to come to your house and give you a mani/pedi.
- Have an old-fashioned sleepover with your best friend.

- Call friends on the phone instead of spending time chatting on Facebook.
- Skype with a faraway friend or family member.
- Read books you read as a child and remember how great it was to be a kid.
- Watch an entire season of your favorite show. Or, spend an entire day watching chick flicks.
- Work on crafts that you don't have time to do normally.
- Do some DIY home improvement projects
- Learn to meditate.
- Catch up on sleep

Tips to Help You Prepare for the Detox

Shopping in advance is a good way to prepare for completing the 3-day detox program.

But if you have never done the detox before there are some other ways that you can prepare too. Using these tips will make the entire 3-days run a lot more smoothly:

- Get a high-quality blender. You are going to need it to blend all the drinks properly. You can buy a small blender very cheaply. A manual juicer, which is very inexpensive, might help with the citrus if you choose drinks containing it.

- Chop the kale. You already know that all the kale will be going into drinks, since there is no solid food eaten on this detox. If you don't chop the kale up into very fine pieces it can clump up in the drinks. Clumped kale is not appetizing at all. Chop all the kale into tiny pieces so that it will break up better in the blender when you are mixing the drinks.

- Drink your detox drinks at the same time each day. Your body's food schedule is going to be way off because of the detox. You may be starving long before you should have another drink, or you may not be hungry at all. Pick times that will be your mealtimes during the detox and stick to those times.

- Leave plenty of time to mix up the drinks. A few recipes call for frozen fruit. Freeze your fresh fruits for the best quality. The drinks contain a lot of ingredients that need to be washed, cut, and prepared. The citrus should be juiced, which is easy with a hand juicer. The liquids need to be measured. All of those steps take time. So start making the drinks about an hour before you want to drink them. If you finish preparation early you can put them in the refrigerator so that they nice and cold.

I hope that you are enjoying this book so far, and if you could spare 30 seconds, I would greatly appreciate you leaving a review on Amazon.com.

Chapter Three

Starting the Detox

Now you are ready to start the detox and start losing weight. Each day of the detox will be the same, so you don't have to worry about trying to keep track of any complicated eating plans.

This will start you on the road to healthy eating habits that will continue after the detox is over.

You will drink the same drinks each day of the weekend, so you can make up batches of one drink at a time and store the extra in the refrigerator.

This may help if you want to make preparing the drinks easier. Just don't store them for more than 3-days. If you have any leftover, throw it out when the detox is over.

Getting Started

Each morning you will start the day with morning detox tea. This can be tough to handle if you're used to starting the day with a cup of coffee because the tea has only trace amounts of caffeine in it.

Ultimately, reducing your caffeine intake will make you feel better.

Morning detox tea is essentially green tea with lemon and some stevia sweetener. The hot green tea will kick start your metabolism and get your body ready to burn fat. You may add matcha, ground ginger or mint leaves to the tea to amp up the detoxifying effects.

Green tea is a metabolism-boosting powerhouse!

In addition to proven weight loss benefits, green tea can help with everything from stress, to liver disorders, to diabetes. While coffee can cause jitters, tea is soothing and relaxing.

It is a pleasant way to start the morning. After the detox is done, you might find that you like starting the day with detox tea.

The tea is all you will have first thing in the morning, but an hour or so later you will have a breakfast drink. This detox has no solid food on it so you will be drinking various types of drinks throughout the weekend but not eating.

If you normally skip breakfast just drinking the tea probably won't be too much of a change for you. But if you ordinarily have a substantial breakfast, you might find it hard to just have tea.

Hang in there! Don't give up when you get hungry. You are supposed to feel hungry during a detox. You are emptying out the body of all the wastes that have built up. Your body is working hard, and that will make you hungry.

However, you already have a powerful hunger-fighting tool in your arsenal!

Green tea contains a substance called epigallocatechin gallate, or EGCG. According to nutritionists, EGCG creates a satisfied feeling when consumed, so your detox tea should help reduce those hunger pangs. Adding a ½ teaspoon of matcha should improve this effect.

Another trick for fighting off hunger is to burn a food scented candle, which can fool your body into thinking that you have eaten more than you have.

Additionally, you can drink as much water as you want. So, whenever you get hungry, drink a bottle of water. Not only will this help you feel full, it will assist in the detox.

The more water you drink, the more impurities and toxins you will flush out of your body. Remember, it will be worth a minor amount of discomfort for a couple of days to look amazing for your event.

Breakfast

An hour or so after drinking the detox tea you can have the breakfast drink. The High-Powered breakfast drink is composed of water, flax seeds, raspberries, banana, spinach, almond butter and lemon. Your other breakfast choices will have similar ingredients. That probably sounds like a crazy combination!

However, these smoothie-like drinks has been carefully calculated by nutritionists to give you the nutrition that you need, and supports your body during the cleansing.

The fiber in the flax seed and the banana will help you feel full so that you do not feel as if you are starving all morning.

This breakfast drink is similar in taste and texture to a normal breakfast smoothie so it won't seem too different from what you might normally drink the morning.

Unlike those smoothies, however, it will give you a powerful nutritional boost that will help your body burn fat and cleanse itself of toxins and bacteria.

If you normally eat a substantial meal, like bacon and eggs, or a bagel for breakfast, the change may be difficult. You might feel as if you have to force yourself to drink your detox drink.

However, you will only be drinking it for 3-days. Also, you will have lost up to 10 pounds by the end of it. Is that not worth the struggle of drinking a smoothie each morning?

Preparing the Drinks

You will have something similar to this for lunch and dinner, so you might want to make the drinks ahead of time in big batches.

If you make a large amount of any drink, you can put it in a pitcher and store it in the fridge for the remainder of the detox. That way you only have to go through the hassle of making each drink once.

After you have your breakfast drink, you will not have another meal drink for a few more hours. You can drink water. At any point on the detox, you can and should drink water.

Remember that it aids in your body functions, and assists the detox process. If you don't want plain water, you can put a tiny amount of lemon juice in your water.

Mid-Morning Vitamin Boost

Around the middle of the morning, you should take half of your multivitamin tablet and the probiotic supplement. You might need to get a pill cutter from the pharmacy in order to cut your vitamin in half. You will be taking half of the multivitamin in the morning and half in the afternoon. This allows your body time to process the vitamins in between drinks, and thus get more nutrition out of them.

It is unimportant if you do not cut it perfectly in half. As long as you are getting the entire vitamin each day, that is the most important thing. Taking your probiotic in the middle of the morning will get your gut working. That will help you lose weight and bring the body back into balance.

Feeling Sick is Normal

You may feel bloated or nauseated when the probiotic first starts to work. If you do, there is no cause for worry. Your body's reaction is totally normal.

Remember that you are cleaning out your systems. So, there is bound to be some discomfort as all that waste gets flushed out of the body. You may find yourself having to go to the bathroom a lot more often over the course of the 3-day detox. That is also normal. Those wastes have to get pushed out of the body so that your body can function better again.

Take it Easy

The first morning will be the hardest because your body will not be used to the cleaning yet. Take it easy and rest a lot. Do not plan on going out and running errands, exercising or doing too much more than just sleeping or simple chores.

On the second and third days, you may want to go out for some light exercise but the first day it is probably a good idea to just stay home, rest, and let your body get used to the detox.

Lunch

When lunchtime rolls around it will be time for another drink. The High-Powered lunchtime drink is made from celery, kale, cucumbers, green apple, lime, pineapple, coconut oil and almond milk. Think of it as a liquid salad with tasty green vegetables and fruit. Your other lunch choices will have similar ingredients.

The oil and almond milk in your lunch drink will provide the fat that your body needs to keep running. Healthy fats like these are good for your body.

Having fat may seem counterproductive, but as previously discussed, your body will crave it to feel full. If you give it healthy fats, you will avoid the temptation of unhealthy ones.

Like your car, your body needs fuel. The food that you eat, or in the case of the detox, the drinks that you drink are your body's fuel. If your body does not get a certain amount of carbs, protein, and healthy fats, it will start to shut down.

If that happens, your body will go into starvation mode, causing it to conserve its resources. So, you will not lose any weight.

Thus, the drinks that you will have on the detox are all carefully planned to provide exactly the ratio of healthy carbs, healthy fats and protein that your body needs to maximize weight loss.

Instead of focusing on the taste of what you are drinking or the meals that you would rather be eating, remind yourself that you are giving your body the fuel that it needs to feel better and look fantastic. The reminder will help you so that you will not feel deprived.

The First Day is the Hardest

By lunchtime on the first day of the detox, you may be ready to throw in the towel. After all, you will be hungry, tired and cranky!

Focus on your goal to help you keep going. Within 24 hours of starting the 3-day detox you will start to notice that you are losing weight even if you don't feel great yet.

By the end of the second day your body will have adjusted a little to the new drinks and it will be burning fat like crazy while flushing out your body.

Once you start to see some amazing results it will be a lot easier to remain motivated and stay on the detox. Success breeds success.

So just stay focused on getting through the first 24 hours. After that, it will be easier than you might think to continue with the detox and become accustomed to drinking all your meals instead of eating.

Mid-Afternoon Vitamin Break

In the middle of the afternoon, it will be time to take the other half of your multivitamin and the Omega 3 fatty acid supplements. Do not skip this step!

During the detox, it is very important that you take the Omega 3 supplement to keep your brain healthy and give it what it needs to keep functioning well.

Snack

Do you usually reach for a snack in the late afternoon? On the 3-day detox you can still have a snack, it just has to be one of the drinks that is already on the plan. You can have any of the drinks that you like, a breakfast, lunch or dinner drink. It's totally up to you.

You may find that on the second or third day you do not even want the snack. The more your body adjusts to the detox diet the more efficient it will be. So, you may not even be hungry in the late afternoon by the second day. It is perfectly acceptable to skip the snack if you are not hungry.

Dinner

The High-Powered dinner drink consists of mango, blueberries, coconut water, kale, lemon, avocado, cayenne pepper and flax seeds. The pepper will give the drink a little kick of flavor but that is not the most important function of the pepper.

Cayenne pepper is an excellent internal cleanser. It will make your body burn more calories and it helps to detoxify the liver. Your liver is the organ that purifies your systems and cleans the toxins out of the blood.

Over time, the liver can start to break down because you have overworked it with an unhealthy diet and lifestyle. Adding a little cayenne or ginger to any of the ginger drinks can charge them up even further! Doing a 3-day detox helps repair your liver and get it functioning the way it should. When the excess waste is gone, your liver will not have to work so hard.

When that happens, you will naturally have an easier time losing weight as the liver processes out fat and unhealthy foods that you have eaten.

Of course, once the detox is over, you should be making an effort to eat a healthier diet so that your liver does not become overwhelmed and suffer from another slowdown. Your new healthier diet will keep you from gaining weight and make sure that your liver does not become sluggish or damaged.

Detox Bath

The detox bath is a lovely way to end the day while you are detoxing. Make your bath an event. Light some candles or incense to help you relax. Mix the Lavender essential oil into the Epsom salts and pour them into a hot bath.

Soak in the tub for at least half an hour. This is the minimum time it will take the Epsom salts to pull impurities out of your skin. Read a book, browse through a magazine, or watch a TV show on your smart phone or tablet. If you want to make the bath a truly spa-like experience, you can give yourself a facial or a pedicure.

You can detox your face with a homemade skin mask. Honey may be spread directly on the skin and left to moisturize and purify until you are ready to leave the bath. It may sound sticky, but honey actually dissolves quickly in warm water, and is an easy mask from a common household ingredient.

Put an eye pillow over your eyes and just rest in the warm water for 30 minutes while your body becomes pure and clean.

Don't Skip the Detox Bath

If you are not a huge fan of baths you may not find the detox bath too appealing. Do it anyway. Toxins will be released through your skin as well as through your body's waste removal system.

Those toxins will clog your pores and build up on your skin unless you get rid of them with a detoxifying bath. The bath will leave your skin glowing and beautiful.

If you don't have a bathtub, you can get the some of the same benefits with a salt scrub in the shower. The bath is the best way to detoxify the skin, so if you have a tub, you should use it. Epsom salts can relieve any bodily aches and pains you develop over the course of the detox, but only if you soak in it.

However, if you don't have a tub you can mix the essential oil into the Epsom salts and then use it like a scrub on your body for a similar detoxifying effect. Don't forget to scrub the soles of your feet and the backs of your arms.

Salt scrubs are good for your skin so you might want to use them a little more often after the 3-day detox. You will already have the Epsom salts and the essential oil so you might as well start giving yourself a detoxifying salt scrub once a week.

Daily Menu for the 3-day Detox

Here's a quick reference layout of what you will be drinking and when during the 3-day detox. Remember to drink your drinks at the same time each day and start preparing them early.

- Wake up with green tea with lemon and stevia
- Breakfast drink

- Mid-Morning vitamin boost with probiotic supplement
- Lunch drink
- Mid-afternoon vitamin boost with Omega 3 supplement
- Snack
- Dinner drink
- Detoxifying bath

For each of the 3-days that you are on the detox, this is the diet you will follow each day.

Even though it might seem restrictive and hard to follow it is not as bad as it seems. The drinks are designed to be more filling than they might at first appear.

Once you get through the first 24 hours, you will think the 3-day detox is comparatively easy. You may even want to do the detox again just to feel healthier after you have finished it.

You may even inspire your family and friends to try it when they see how great you look. You could make it a monthly event with your friends to detox one weekend so that you all look great and feel great too. Having the support of a friend or relative who is going through the 3-day detox with you can only encourage you.

Chapter Four

What You're Drinking

The drinks that you will be drinking in place of meals on the 3-day detox are all made from fresh fruit and vegetables with a few healthy oils thrown in. The breakfast drink and dinner drink have flax seeds also, which add some fiber to the drink.

Why were these particular ingredients chosen? The properties of these fruits and vegetables offer a clue. You have already learned about green tea and the effect it has on your metabolism.

What are some of the specific ways in which the foods in your drinks help your 3-day detox? Many are called "super foods".

Why? Raspberries contain ketones, which speed up the metabolism, and help prevent fat from being absorbed by the body.

Strawberries contain phytonutrients, which have anti-inflammatory and antioxidant properties.

Almonds contain concentrated nutrition and healthy fats; hence they are included in your detox drinks in the form of butter and milk.

Blueberries contain antioxidants, which fight free radical buildup. Free radicals are just one of the toxins mucking up your systems.

It is common knowledge that bananas are an excellent source of potassium, which protects your blood vessels from damage. Additionally, the texture of the banana makes the drinks more filling.

Spinach, which is packed with nutrients, also contains a newly discovered phytonutrient that helps protect the digestive track from damage. Other greens have similar nutritional properties.

Flax seeds, in addition to adding fiber to your drinks, have been shown to reduce cancer risk, heart disease, and the danger of diet induced diabetes.

Lemon is a blood purifier, bolsters the immune system, and treats infections. Other citrus fruits have similar properties.

Celery is an anti-inflammatory agent and a further source of antioxidants.

Kale, that currently trendy green, is power packed with more vitamins and minerals than other greens.

Cucumbers contain antioxidants, and also fight heart disease and inflammation.

Everyone knows an apple a day keeps the doctor away. Why? They are loaded with nutrition and can improve neurological health and prevent dementia.

Coconut oil contains healthy fat, and has been linked by some people to thyroid health and a boosted immune system.

Mangoes contain many needed vitamins and minerals.

Avocadoes contain over 20 vitamins and minerals per serving, and provide healthy fat and fiber.

Turmeric contains bioactive compounds, including curcumin, which have a variety of satisfactory effects on the body, such as the detoxifying of antioxidants, controlling inflammation, reducing heart disease, treating depression, preventing certain types of cancer, fighting the signs and damage of aging, and even preventing Alzheimer's Disease.

Parsley contains Vitamins A, B 12, C and K. It has anti-inflammatory, and antioxidant properties, lowers blood pressure, relaxes stiff muscles, aids in digestion, and may help prevent and fight some forms of cancer.

Ginger's anti-nausea effects are well known, but it has many more benefits. It has a broad spectrum of antibacterial, antiviral, antioxidant, and anti-parasitic. It has been shown to help arthritis better than over the counter medication with few side effects, and it can help tired muscles and cramps.

Cinnamon mimics sweetness, and helps you feel full. In addition to all of the antioxidant benefits we have discussed above, , like heart health, and sugar regulation, cinnamon can protect against Parkinson's disease.

Honey is a natural miracle. It can be used on the skin for wound healing, having antiseptic and antibacterial properties, and is so useful that pharmaceutical companies have created Medihoney.

Your local honey has these same healing properties. Additionally, local honey as food can fight airborne allergens. It can ease the early symptoms of a cold and has been found as effective, if not, more so than over the counter cough remedies. It may help ease stomach complaints as well.

The research on these "super foods" is voluminous, and scientists are still studying and learning more. Each nutritional element of your drinks has been well thought out by nutritionists, and planned to give you the maximum results on your 3-day detox.

Substitutions

You can play with the ratios in these drinks to make them more to your taste. If you like them a little thicker you can add a little less water, although you should be drinking as much water as possible.

Stick to the recommended amount of fruits and vegetables in order to keep the combinations in the drink balanced. However, if you find that you really dislike one ingredient or another you can substitute a comparable fruit or vegetable. Try to choose one with similar properties.

Preparing the Fruits and Vegetables

You may have to spend more time than you imagine washing and chopping the ingredients for the drinks. Fresh food and whole food does require a little bit of preparation. Still, ultimately it is worth it.

To get the fruits and vegetables ready for your 3-day detox first clean the sink. Then rinse the fruits and vegetables. Put the stopper in the sink and fill the sink with warm water and some vinegar. Let the fruits and vegetables soak in the vinegar water.

The vinegar in the water will kill any bacteria on the fruits and vegetables. It will also help them stay fresh longer. Cleaning berries in a vinegar bath will keep them from molding.

After the fruits and vegetables have soaked for about 30 minutes, you can pull the stopper from the sink and rinse them with clean water. Let them dry and then you can peel and chop them if they need it.

It's also a good idea to take a little extra time and chop up the fruits and vegetables so that they are in tiny pieces. That way they will break down totally in the blender and you won't end up with chewy pieces in your drink. No one wants to drink a meal full of large bits of kale or chunks of fruit.

How to Make the Drinks

You can change these a little bit to make them taste better to you but try to stick to this list as much as possible. They were designed to help you detox most efficiently, so try and keep the proportions essentially the same. You'll have a choice of several drinks for each meal, so one of them is bound to sound tasty to you!

Once again, thank you for reading this book, and I hope you're getting a lot of valuable information. I would greatly appreciate it if you could take 30 seconds to leave me a review for this book on Amazon.com.

Breakfast Drinks

High Powered Detox Drink

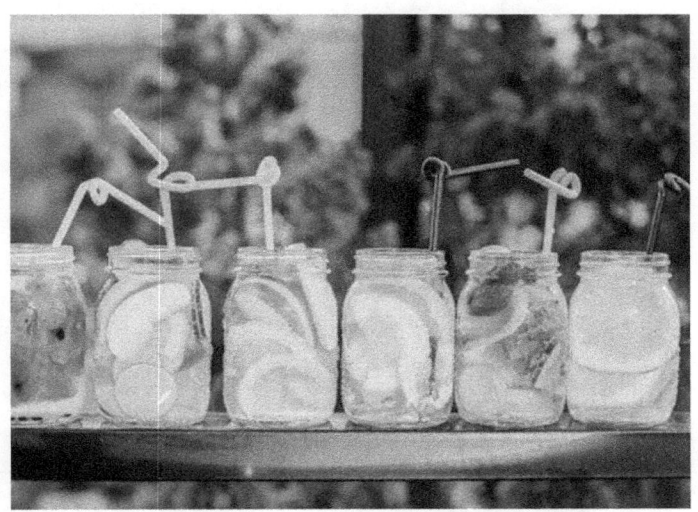

Ingredients

- 1 cup water
- 1 tablespoon of ground flax seed
- 1 cup raspberries
- 1 banana
- ¼ cup spinach
- 1 tablespoon almond butter
- 2 teaspoons lemon juice or lemon zest

Method

1. Blend until it has a milkshake like consistency.

Detox Blueberry Fruit Smoothie

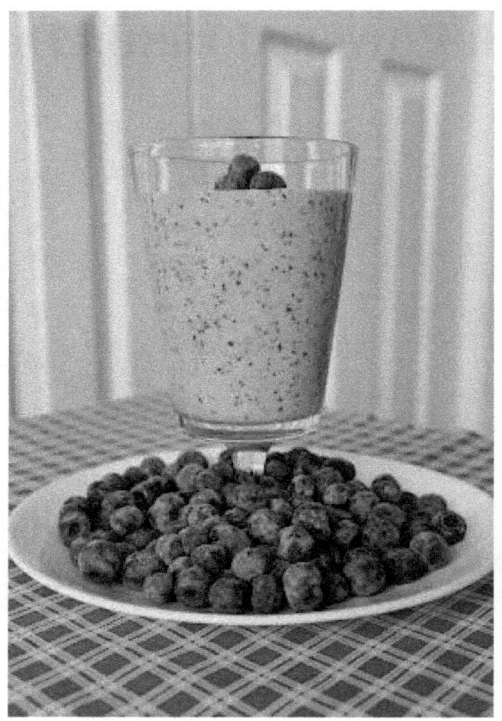

Ingredients

- ½ cup frozen blueberries
- ¼ cup unsweetened cranberry juice
- 1 or 2 bananas (to taste)

Method

1. Blend into a smoothie-like consistency.

Orange Surprise

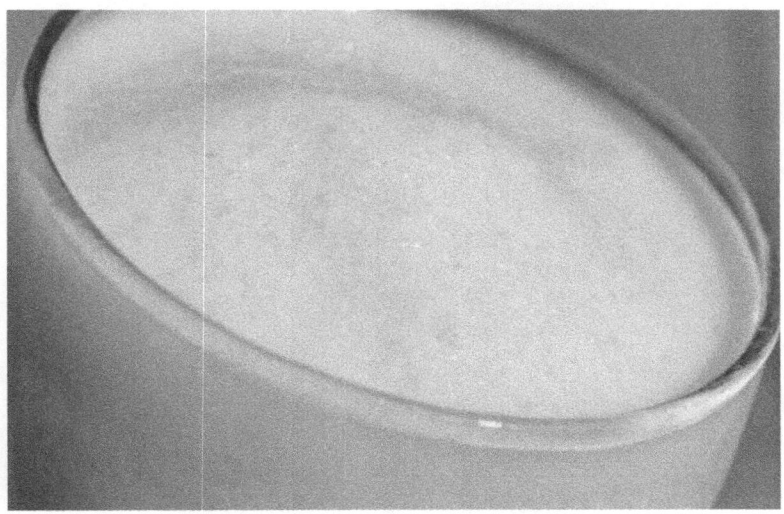

Ingredients

- 2 apples, quartered
- 2 medium carrots, chunked
- 1 stalk celery, chunked
- Juice of 4-5 calamansi limes

Method

1. If you have a juicer, you won't need to juice the limes separately. If you are blending, juice the limes, and then blend ingredients as finely as possible.

Mango Ginger Lemonade

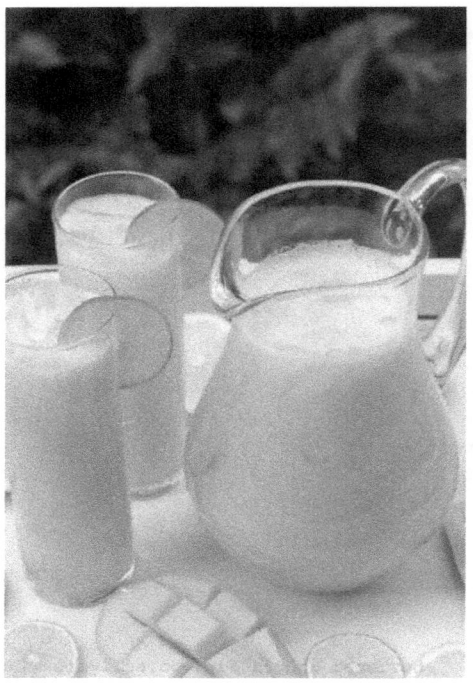

Ingredients

- ½ a mango
- 1 lemon
- 1 thin slice ginger
- Zest of 1 lemon
- 3 to 4 ice cubes

Method

1. Blend all the ingredients finely.

Super Green Detox Smoothie

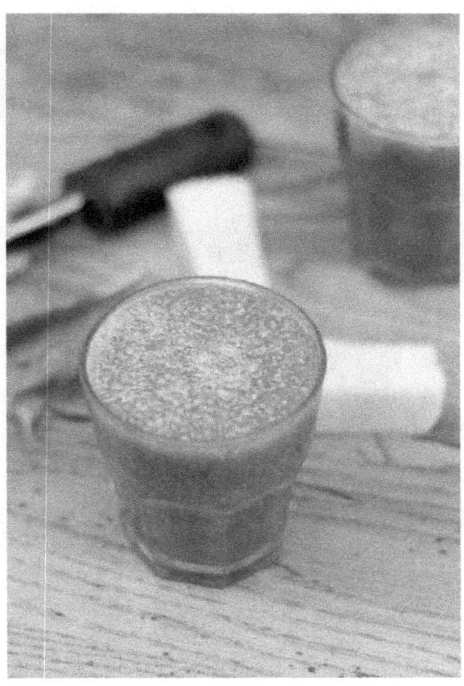

Ingredients

- 1 ¼ cups pineapple juice
- Juice from ¼ of a lemon
- A Handful of fresh spinach leaves
- ¼ teaspoon of freshly grated ginger

Method

1. Grate the ginger. Combine all ingredients. Blend until liquefied and green.

Carrot Apple Ginger Smoothie

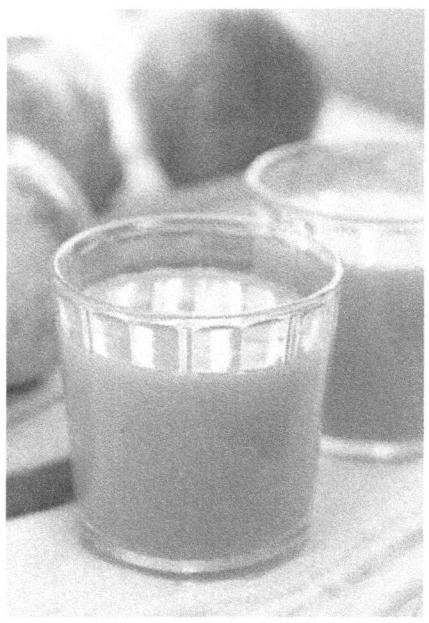

Ingredients

- 1 teaspoon flax seeds
- 1 red apple, peeled
- 8 baby carrots
- ¼ inch nub of ginger root, skin removed (should be moist)
- 1 cup lukewarm water

Method

1. The flax seeds must soak for 30 minutes in the lukewarm water to create flax seed water.

2. You will know the process is complete when there is a film floating on top of the water, and the seeds have turned gooey.

3. After you have created flax seed water, combine all the ingredients and blend to a smoothie-like consistency.

Cranberry Bliss Smoothie

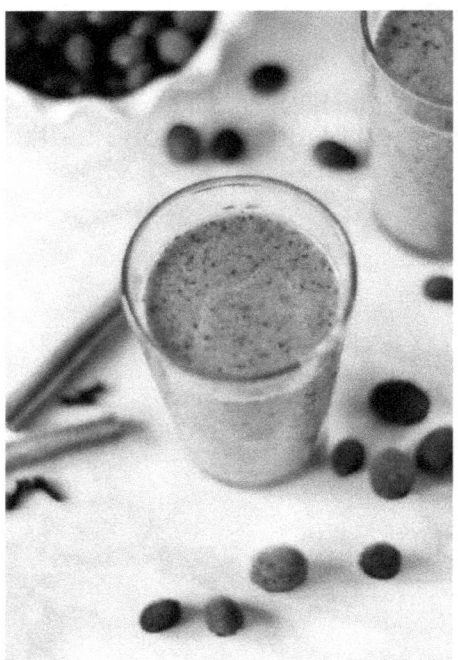

Ingredients

- 1 apple, quartered with peel on
- 1 pear, quartered with peel on
- ½ lemon, remove peel and seeds
- ½ cup fresh cranberries
- 1 cup water
- 2 to 3 ice cubes
- 2 teaspoons honey
- ½ teaspoon cinnamon
- ½ teaspoon nutmeg
- ½ teaspoon turmeric

Method

1. Blend water and ice. Put in spices, and blend again. Then introduce fruits and honey, blending till it becomes a smoothie-like consistency.

Matcha Mango Pineapple Smoothie

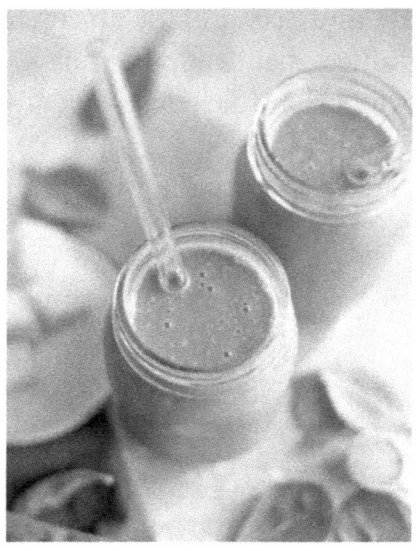

Ingredients

- 1 ¼ teaspoon matcha green tea powder
- 2 teaspoons honey
- 1 cup mango chunks
- 1 tablespoon pineapple juice
- 1 cup pineapple
- ½ cup water
- 2 ice cubes

Method

1. Blend water, ice, and matcha. Then add fruit and juice. Blend until liquefied.

Berry Breakfast

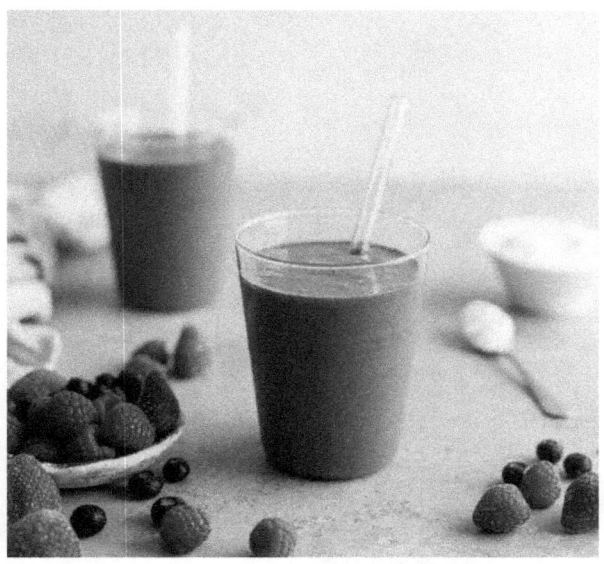

Ingredients

- ½ cup frozen, unsweetened raspberries
- ½ cup unsweetened almond milk
- ¼ cup frozen, pitted cherries
- 2 teaspoons honey
- 1 teaspoon finely grated fresh ginger
- ½ teaspoon ground flax seed
- 1 to 2 teaspoons lemon juice

Method

1. Combine all ingredients in your blender. Puree until smooth.

Morning Glorious

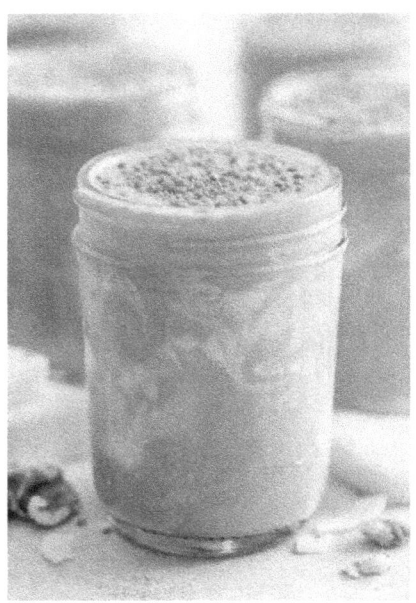

Ingredients

- 1 large cucumber
- A fistful of kale
- A fistful of romaine
- 2 to 3 stalks of celery
- 1 large broccoli stem
- 1 green apple, quartered
- ½ lemon, peeled and quartered

Method

1. Combine all ingredients and puree until smooth.

Lunch Drinks

Here are some delicious lunch choices.

High Powered Lunch Drink

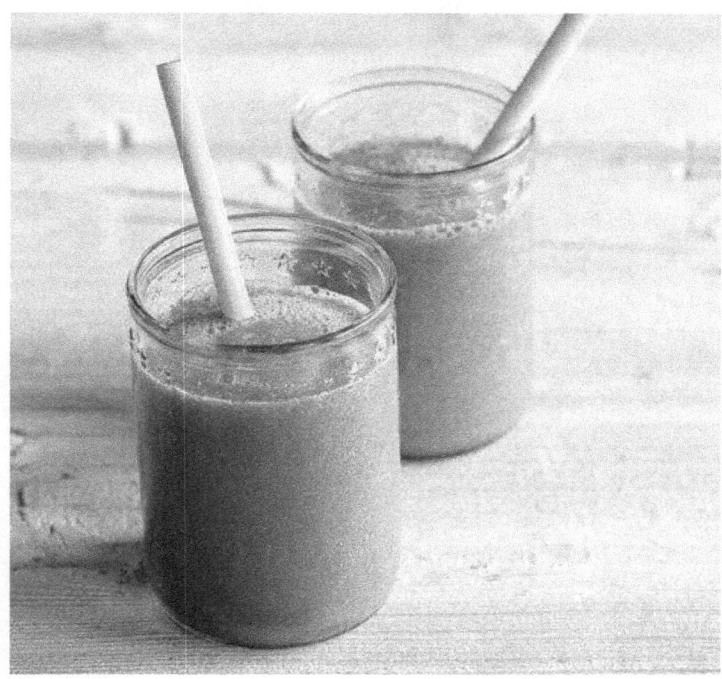

Ingredients

- 4 celery stalks
- 1 cucumber, peeled and seeded or use a seedless cucumber
- 1 cup kale leaves
- ½ cup green apple, peeled
- ½ lime

- 1 Tablespoon of coconut oil
- ½ cup almond milk
- 1 cup of pineapple

Method

1. Combine in your blender and puree.

Smooth Operator

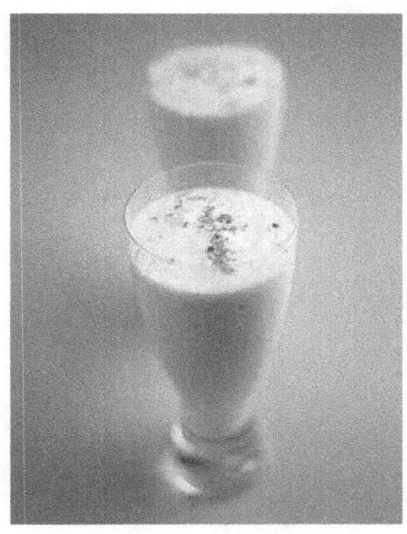

Ingredients

- Fistful of romaine
- ½ Granny Smith apple
- ¼ avocado
- ½ cucumber
- ½ cup jicama
- Handful of cilantro
- 1 lime
- 1 date

Method

1. Combine all ingredients in your blender, and blend into a smoothie-like texture.

Alkalinity Bliss

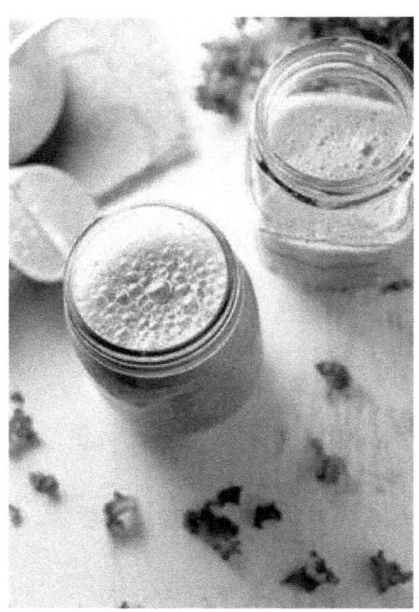

Ingredients

- ¼ avocado
- ½ pear
- ¼ cup coconut water
- 1 packed cup spinach
- 1 cup almond milk
- 1 tsp chia seeds
- ½ cup water

Method

1. Combine all ingredients in your blender and puree.

Hale to the Kale

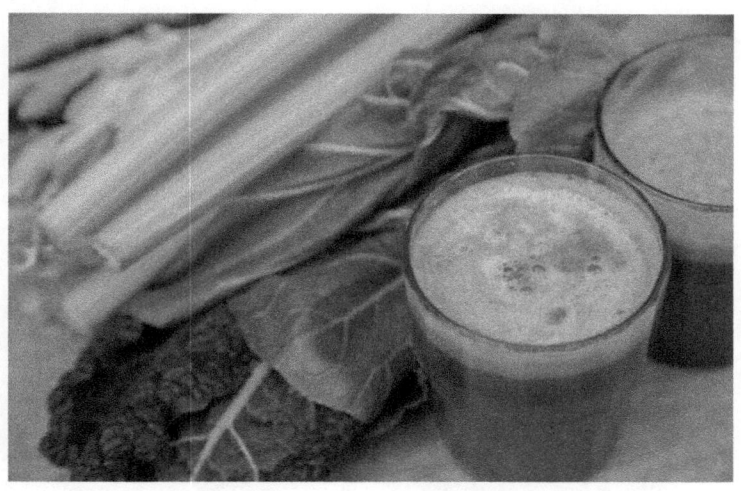

Ingredients

- ½ pear
- ¼ avocado
- ½ cucumber
- ½ lemon
- Handful of cilantro
- 1 packed cup of kale
- ½ inch of ginger
- ½ cup of coconut water
- ½ cup water

Method

1. Chop kale finely. Combine all ingredients and blend.

The Super Green

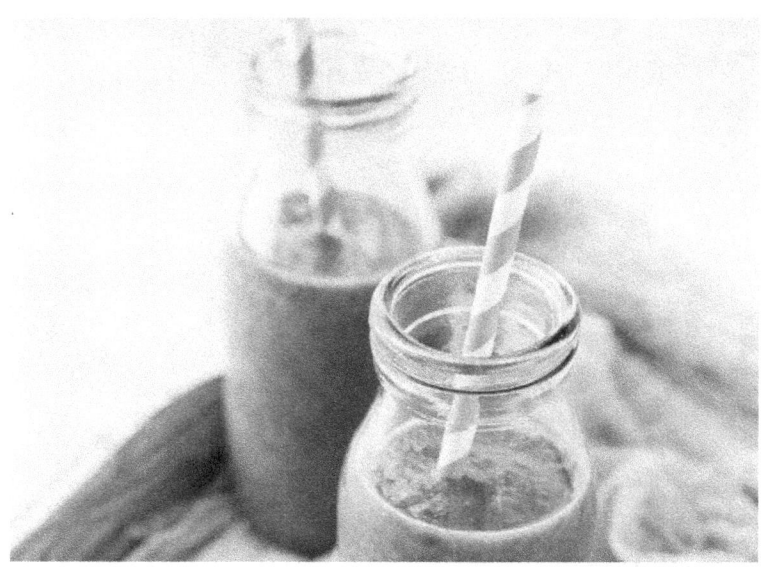

Ingredients

- 1¼ cup finely chopped kale
- 1¼ cup frozen cubed mango
- 1 cup chilled fresh orange juice
- ¼ cup chopped fresh parsley
- ¼ cup chopped fresh mint
- 2 stalks celery

Method

1. Combine all your ingredients in your blender. Puree until smooth.

Strawberry Fields

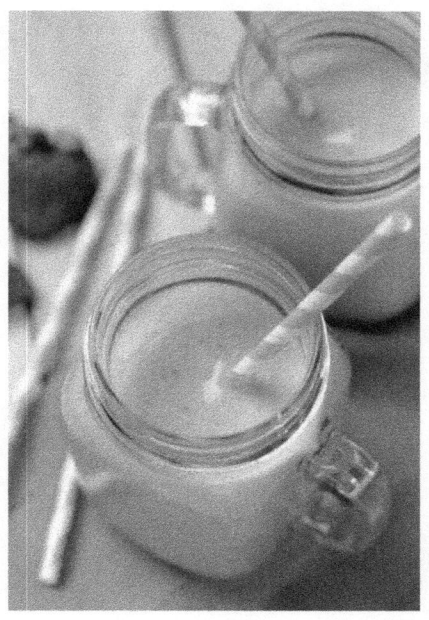

Ingredients

- 1 ½ cups almond milk
- 1 ½ fresh strawberries
- 1 tablespoon lemon zest
- 1 small orange, peeled
- 1 banana
- 1 cup spinach, loosely packed

Method

1. Combine all ingredients in your blender. Blend on high speed until smooth.

The Sicilian

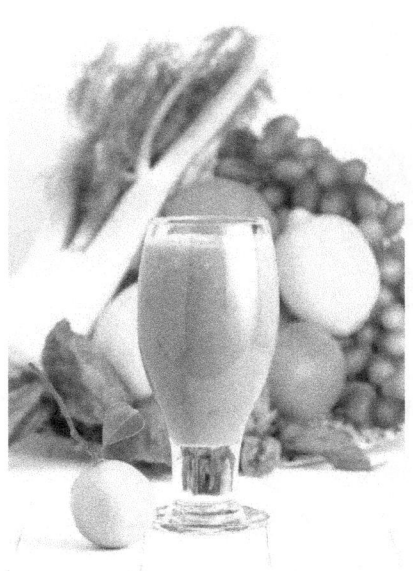

Ingredients

- 3 carrots
- 1 large tomato
- 1 red bell pepper
- 2 cloves garlic
- 2 stalks of celery
- ½ cup watercress
- ½ cup loosely packed spinach

Method

1. Chop vegetables finely. Puree until the drink is a smoothie-like consistency.

Green Machine

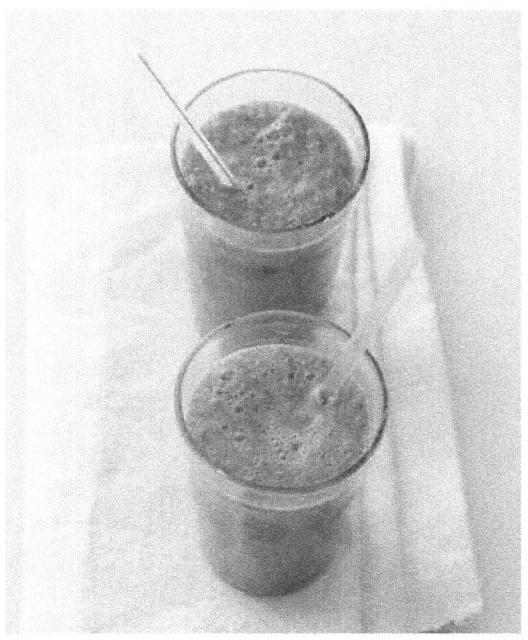

Ingredients

- 1 green apple
- 1 lemon
- 1 cucumber, peeled
- 3 to 4 leaves red leaf lettuce
- ¼ cup mango

Method

1. Blend on high speed to obtain a smoothie-like consistency.

Berry Elixir

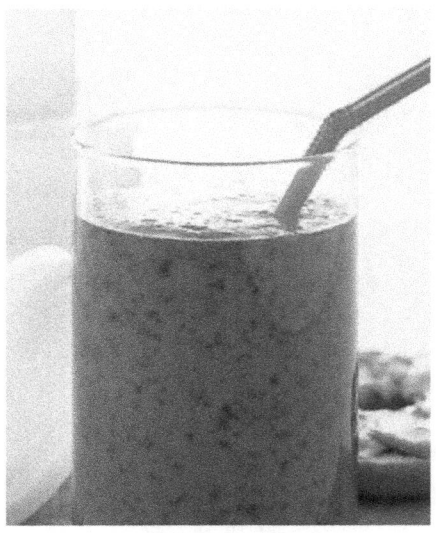

Ingredients

- 1 cup almond milk
- 1 cup blueberries
- ½ cup raspberries
- ½ cup blackberries
- 2 tablespoons Goji berries (soaked for 15 minutes)
- 1 tablespoon coconut oil
- 1 tablespoon ground flaxseed
- 2 dates, pitted

Method

1. Combine all ingredients in your blender and blend until smooth.

Cranberry Cleanser

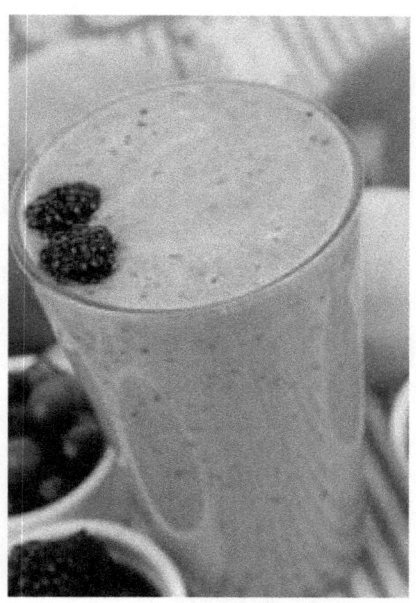

Ingredients

- ½ cup cranberries
- 1 celery stalk
- 1 cucumber
- 1 apple
- 1 pear
- Handful of spinach
- ½ cup water

Method

1. Blend at high speed until smooth.

Dinner Drinks

When it is dinner time, you can check out one of these delectable drinks!

High Powered Dinner Drink

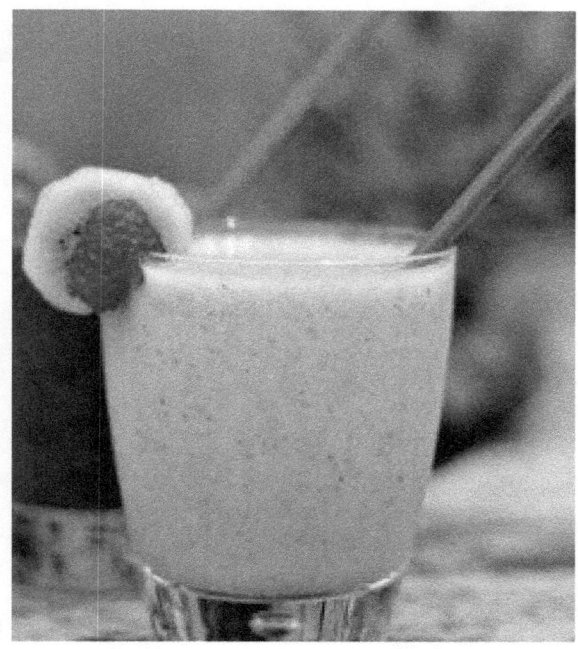

Ingredients

- ½ cup mango
- 1 cup blueberries
- 1 and ½ cups coconut water
- 1 cup kale
- 1Tbsp lemon juice
- ¼ avocado

- ½ Tsp. cayenne pepper
- 1 Tbsp. flax seed

Method

1. Blend all ingredients together until they attain a milkshake-like texture.

Vitamin C Smoothie

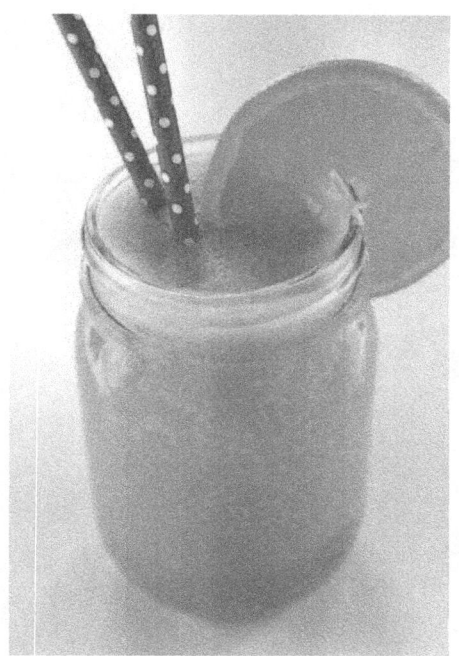

Ingredients

- 2 oranges
- ½ cantaloupe
- 1 tomato
- 1 cup strawberries
- 3 ice cubes

Method

1. Juice the orange. Combine all the ingredients in your blender and puree until smooth.

Vitamin Cocktail

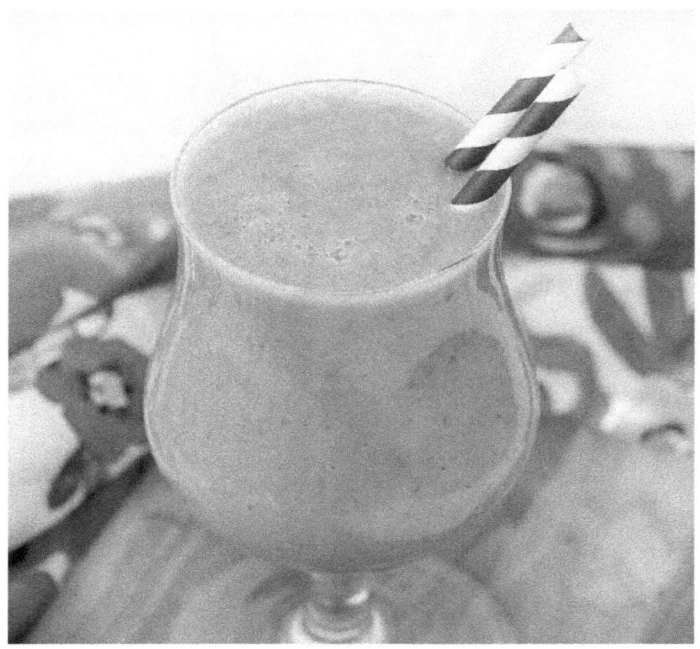

Ingredients

- 1 cup papaya
- ½ cup kale
- ½ cup spinach
- ½ banana
- ½ green apple

Method

1. Blend combined ingredients at high speed until they are a smoothie-like consistency.

Berry Bliss Cocktail

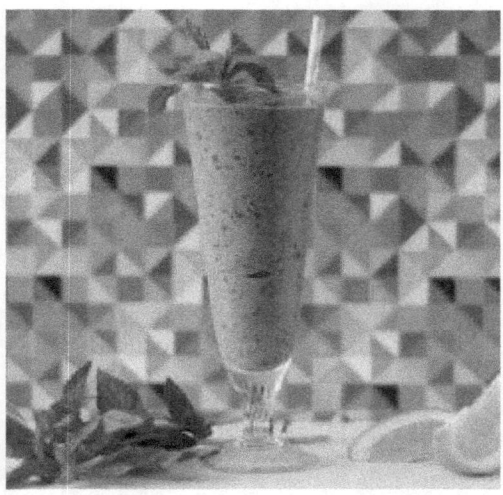

Ingredients

- ¼ cup blueberries
- ¼ cup strawberries
- ¼ raspberries
- ¼ cup kale
- ½ cup water
- 4 ice cubes

Method

1. Place all ingredients into your blender, and pulverize them on high speed.

Green and Glowing Smoothie

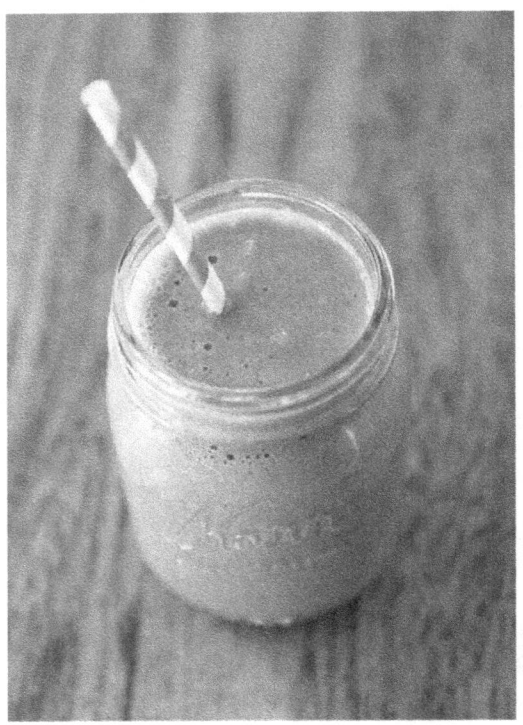

Ingredients

- 1 cup kale, tightly packed
- 1 cup spinach, tightly packed
- 1 pear, quartered, with core removed
- 1 orange, peeled
- 1 banana, peeled
- 1 teaspoon ground flax seeds
- ½ cup water
- 2 cups ice

Method

1. Combine in your blender. Start on low, blend for 30 seconds, move to medium for 30 seconds, then move to high speed until the mixture is completely blended.

Rippled Raspberry Smoothie

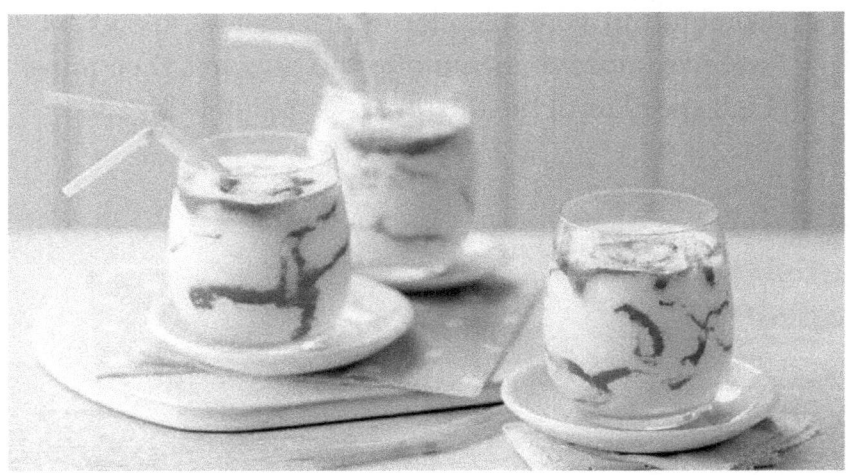

Ingredients

- 1 cups water
- ½ cup almond milk
- ¼ cup dates
- 1 cup raspberries
- 1 cup spinach, loosely packed

Method

1. Combine water, milk and spinach first, blend. Then add fruit, puree until smooth.

Almond Pear Greenie

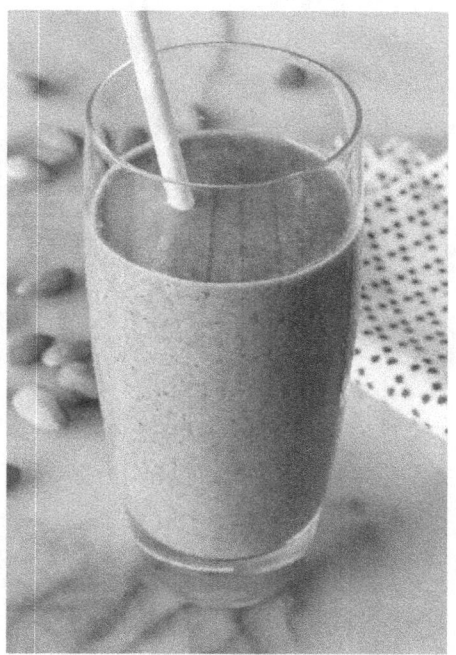

Ingredients

- 1 cup almond milk
- 2 pears, quartered and cored
- ¼ cup almonds
- 1 cup kale, loosely packed

Method

1. Blend liquid and kale. Then add fruit, continue blending at high speed until the mixture attains a smoothie-like texture.

Cool Breeze Mint and Pineapple Smoothie

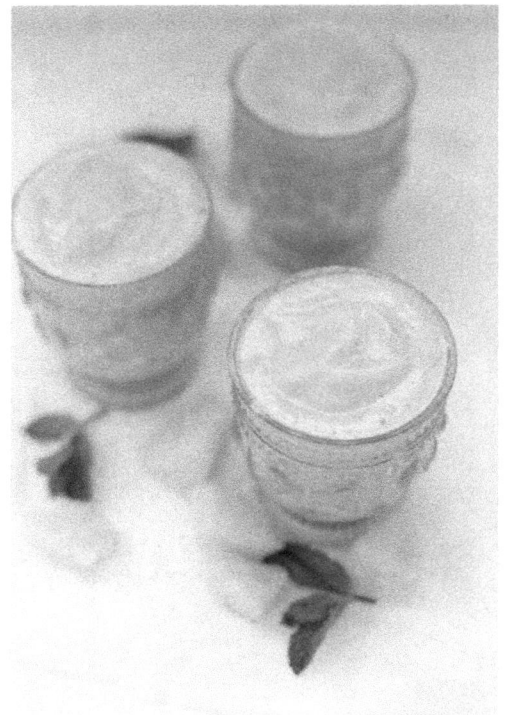

Ingredients

- ½ cup water
- 2 cups pineapple
- 1 banana
- 5 mint leaves
- 1 tablespoon ground flax seeds
- 1 cup spinach
- ½ cup ice

Method

1. Add liquid and spinach to blender, blend thoroughly, then add fruit and flax seeds. Continue blending. Add ice, blend until smooth.

Vitamin Powerhouse Vegetable Smoothie

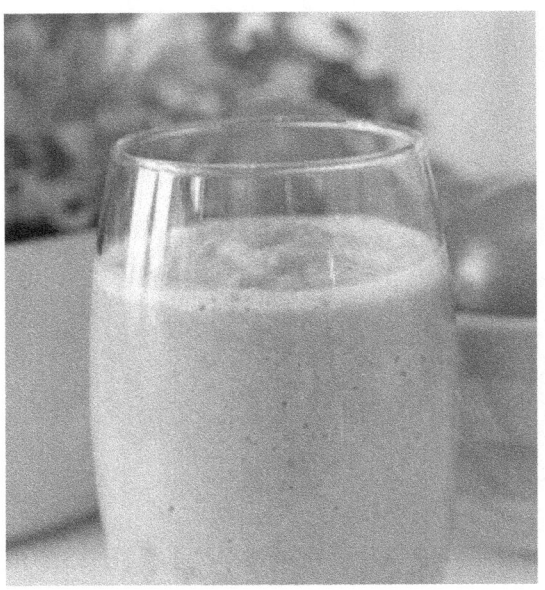

Ingredients

- 1 tomato
- ½ cucumber
- ½ clove garlic
- 1 celery stalk
- 2 cups romaine, loosely packed
- ½ cup avocado
- ¼ teaspoon turmeric
- ½ lemon, peeled and seeded
- 20 mint leaves
- 1 small handful parsley
- 1 teaspoon grated ginger

- 1 pinch cayenne pepper
- 1 cup ice

Method

1. Blend tomato, cucumber, and lemon. Add other ingredients one at a time, blending between each.

2. You may need to add a touch of water, but the tomato, cucumber and lemon are intended to provide enough liquid to enable the mixture to be blended.

3. Once all ingredients are added, add ice and continue to blend until smooth.

Cilantro with Spinach Smoothie

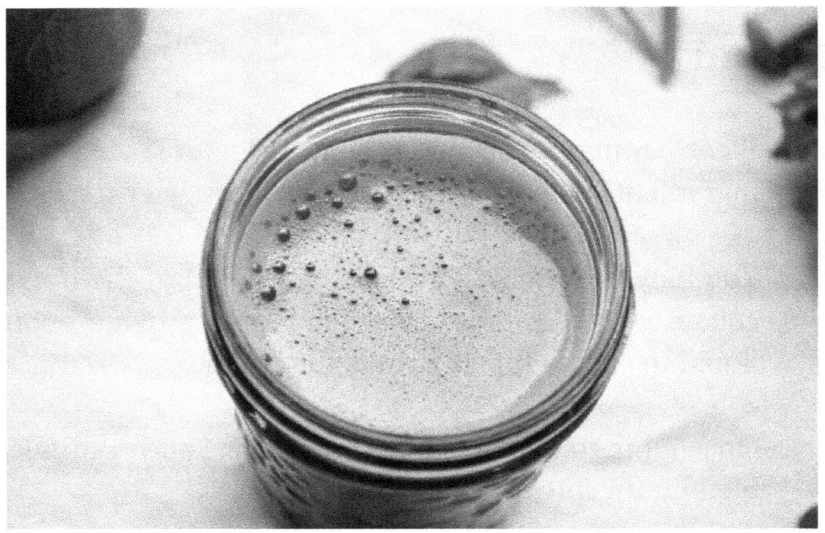

Ingredients

- ¼ cup cilantro
- 1 ½ cup spinach
- 3 bananas
- 1 peeled lime
- 1 inch fresh ginger
- 1 cup water
- 3 ice cubes

Method

1. Add cilantro, spinach, and water to blender. Blend completely, then add fruit and ginger. Continue blending. Add ice. Blend thoroughly

2. What a variety of drink choices! These tasty drinks will help you lose weight and get your body back to burning calories and removing waste the way it should.

3. You may even find that after eating delicious raw foods for 3 whole days you want to keep eating them, especially now that you know all of the benefits. Most of the time people who do well on the 3-day detox start incorporating some of these healthy foods into their regular diet when the detox is over.

4. Adding some of these foods to your regular diet will help you maintain a healthy weight and keep you in good physical shape for the rest of your life.

If you're enjoying this book and would love to let other potential readers know how great it is, please take a few seconds to leave a review on Amazon.com.

Enjoying this book?

Check out my other best sellers!

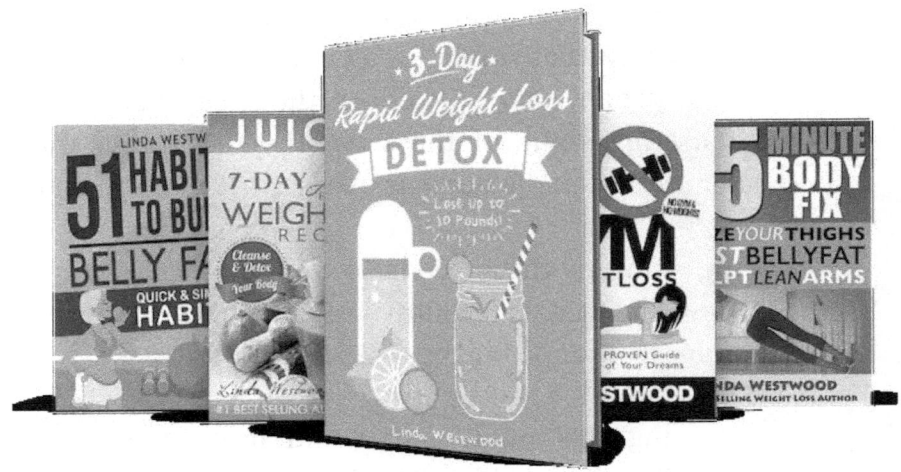

Get your next book on sale here:

TopFitnessAdvice.com/go/books

Chapter Five

Lose Up To 10 Pounds!

The 3-day detox is one of the only ways that you can drop up to 10 pounds in just a few days. It may be somewhat difficult, but it is effective. 10 pounds is about the same as one dress size or pants size. That's why the 3-day detox program is the ideal regimen to do if you have a special event coming up, like a vacation or a wedding.

Dropping up to an entire dress size will give you the confidence that you need to have a great time at the event. You will be sure that you look great.

Even if you don't have a special event coming and you just want to give your body a fresh start, the 3-day detox will help you. By balancing the bacteria in the gut and flushing toxins out of your body, you can lose inches as well as pounds.

Top Detox Tips to Lose More Weight

Exercise and the 3-day Detox

When you first start the detox, you probably won't feel much like exercising. By the second day, you will feel better but you should avoid any strenuous exercises.

During the detox period, your body is going to be working hard already cleaning up and burning fat. Because you will be only drinking meals and not eating, the electrolyte balance in your body can become unbalanced if you are sweating heavily as you would from extensive exercise.

However, light exercise is a great thing idea for day 2 and 3. Walking, swimming, bike riding, yoga, and Pilates are gentle exercises that will help you lose weight during the detox. Just make sure that the exercises you choose are gentle and not stressful.

After the 3-day Detox

When the detox is done and you have lost a large amount of weight, regular exercise will help you keep that weight off. If you continue to eat healthy foods and exercise, you should not have any problem maintaining your weight or even continuing to lose if need be.

If for some reason you do gain back some of the weight that you lost, you can always do the 3-day detox again. Some people choose to do the detox on a regular basis just to help maintain their current weight.

Twist Your Way

We have talked about light exercise, of course, but serious yoga practitioners have claimed that certain twisting postures assist in releasing toxins, helping you speed up the detox/weight loss process.

So add these moves to your exercise routine. You should be able to find demonstrations of these poses on-line:

- Bharadvaja's Twist
- Half Lord of the Fishes Pose
- Marichi's Pose
- Noose Pos
- Revolved Head to Knee Pose
- Revolved Side Angle Pose
- Revolved Triangle Pose
- Twisting Triangle

Purge Your Pantry

Take this time at home to clean out your cabinets and refrigerator of any unhealthy foods and get rid of them. If you are committed to changing your lifestyle, you should rid yourself of temptation, not just for the period of the 3-day detox, but for always. You are getting over your addiction to junk food.

Are you going to give yourself fuel for bad habits to return? You know what you should be eating, even when you return to eating solid food. If it is not on your healthy eating plan, it has to go. If it is refrigerated, trash it. If not, box it up. When you are finished with your detox you could take it to a food bank.

Combat Cravings

Cravings can cause you to slip and sabotage your 3-day detox. So try some of these tips to fight the urges.

When hunger strikes, clench your fists! Tensing any muscle and holding it for 30 seconds is helpful in regaining your focus. Also, pick a new activity, quickly. Distracting yourself is very important when cravings begin, so stop what you are doing and chose a short activity, like painting your nails. Usually ten minutes are long enough to allow those cravings to pass.

Do some deep breathing. Focus on your breathing for some cleansing breaths. Count to 5 as you breathe in and then again when you breathe out. Do this 20 to 30 times, and the craving will pass.

Focus on the Future

Spend some of your time thinking about the things that will change due to your new, healthy lifestyle.

Not about what you may perceive as negative changes, but the reasons why you wanted to lose weight in the first place. If your reason was to go to an event, imagine yourself there, looking amazing.

Imagine the compliments from friends on how great you look. Picture telling them all about your 3-day detox, about your plans for a new healthy life. The power of positive thinking is real!

Make a list of things you'll be able to do that you couldn't when you were unhealthy. Start planning how to actually get out and do them.

The more thoughts you focus on the new slimmer you, the more you will help your weight loss.

Make a Plan

It may help you to focus on your ultimate goal of a healthy lifestyle, to stick to your detox through its conclusion.

There are some eating plans listed below. Think about how you live and eat normally, and try and pick a plan you can stick with, and changes you want to make that you feel like are feasible.

Your success with the 3-day detox is intended to lead you to a healthier life, and when you stick with your plan, and have even more success, it will inspire you to bigger changes.

Chapter Six

Be Safe

Doing any kind of detox is going to be tough on the body. It is important that you make safety a priority during the 3-day detox. The liquid diet may seem extreme, but really that is what the body needs in order to fully cleanse itself.

The detox is safe, provided you observe a few precautions. Moreover, you need to understand and prepare for what really happens during the detox process.

Removing Toxins is a Mess

The fat and toxins that your body is losing during a detox can cause some uncomfortable physical symptoms. Laying low during the detox will make it easier to manage the side effects of the detox process. It can get messy to rid your body of so much waste all at once.

What to Expect

When you are on a detox you are radically shifting your diet. This can affect your blood sugar which can cause side effects. Even if you are taking a good multivitamin and a good probiotic, you can expect to have some physical symptoms like:

- Gas
- Bloating

- Nausea
- Fatigue
- Fuzzy thinking
- Sleeplessness
- Restless sleep
- Irritability
- Headache
- Constipation
- Diarrhea
- Flu like symptoms
- General aches and pains
- Body odor
- Itchy skin
- Bad breath

All of these symptoms are within the realm of possibility, but they will go away when the detox is done. However, until then you will need to find ways to manage them so that your body can detox safely.

Here are some tips to help you manage the unpleasant side effects of a detox:

Get More Sleep

Sleep is even more important during a detox than it normally is. If you are tired, sleep.

Sleep is the best thing to do while you detox. Take naps and let your body rest itself. Make plenty of time to relax throughout the 3-days. This is one time that it is ok to spend 3-days on the couch or in bed with books and TV.

Hydrate Hydrate Hydrate

Drink at least six to eight glasses of water each day. Regular hydration is essential to good health, and never more so than during the 3-day detox. You will be losing water very quickly as your body sheds toxins and you need to replace that water to be sure your body keeps functioning.

Throughout the detox you should be drinking as much water as you can. You can flavor the water with a little lemon juice or you can drink hot green tea. Just don't put any sweetener in the tea. The more water you drink the faster the toxins will get flushed out of your body.

Keep a Detox Journal

Keep track of your side effects and bodily reactions. In order to track if a symptom is getting worse you should write them all down.

Keep a detox journal that documents the different side effects of the detox. Write down any problems or side effects that you think are related to the detox.

Sweat Those Toxins Out

Turn the heat up. Heat will help draw the toxins out of your body. That's why a hot bath is part of the detox.

Turn the heat up so that you can release those toxins a little faster. Hydration must be stressed again for just this reason.

What You Need to Watch Out For

The 3-day detox may be slightly unpleasant, but if it starts to become extremely uncomfortable you might need to get checked out by a doctor. Throughout the detox process stay in touch with friends and family. Because the detox diet can be a little hard on the body, it is a good idea to check in with them regularly.

A follow up to this: make it part of your plan to get in touch with a certain person, who will then check on you if they do not hear from you.

If you start to notice any of these symptoms, you should visit your primary physician for a thorough examination before finishing the detox:

- Fever
- Extreme nausea
- Extreme sweating
- Disorientation
- Excessive vomiting
- Trouble concentrating
- Forgetting information like your name
- Confusion
- Fainting
- Extreme fatigue
- Extreme weight loss such as losing 20+ pounds

You can see why it might be a good idea to have a detox buddy who will check on you if you fail to get in touch with him or her.

Although serious problems are rare, they can occur. If you notice any of these side effects, or if your symptoms seem debilitating, then get checked out by a doctor immediately. You can always go back and do the detox again once you are cleared by a physician to do so.

Others who are considering purchasing this book would love to know what you think. If you could spare a few seconds, they would greatly appreciate reading an honest review from you. Simply visit the page on Amazon.com.

Chapter Seven

Next Weekend

You can use the 3-day detox as a chance to start living a healthier life. Take advantage of the fact that your body has been cleansed of years of toxins and bad food choices. After you have lost up to ten pounds on the detox, you will not want to stop losing weight and feeling incredible.

Healthy Eating

One of the reasons why the detox works so well is because you are eating nothing but fresh and whole foods for 3-days. The fact that they are in a liquid form doesn't matter. What does matter is that you are getting top of the line nutrition from the best possible source. If you want to keep looking and feeling great you need to keep eating healthy.

Information on what you should be eating is widely available, and any of the foods that have gone into your detox drinks would be excellent choices.

The single most important tip on healthy eating is this: learn what the portion size is, and stick to that.

Liquid Diets

If you have a lot of weight to lose you may want to consider a liquid diet after you have done the 3-day detox. Liquid diets can be very effective for weight loss.

However, do not continue the detox diet longer than 3-days without consulting your physician. Liquid diets need to be carefully supervised by a doctor to be sure that you are getting all the vitamins and minerals that you need to stay healthy while you lose weight.

If you like the success that comes from a liquid diet but you don't want to go on an all liquid diet, you can do a hybrid diet. You can eat one or two small meals each day and have some of the 3-day detox meal drinks during the rest of the day.

A hybrid diet will give you the nutrition that you need and the weight loss that you want. If you like the meal drinks that are used in the 3-day detox you can easily substitute them for meals at any time.

Sometimes you might want to drop a few pounds without doing a full detox. Drinking meal drinks for just a day can give you the results you want without you having to spend 3-days doing a full detox.

Losing the Taste for Junk Food

Even if you are a hard-core fan of junk food, chocolate, and high calorie foods you will find that after the detox they do not taste good to you anymore.

More than once someone who has done the 3-day detox celebrates with a bag of chips or a chocolate bar and ends up throwing the treat away because it tastes terrible now that they have detoxed from processed food. That is because once your body gets rid of the toxic remnants of those foods you will not crave them anymore, and they will taste good to you when you eat them.

You will be shocked by how differently your body receives them. Before the detox, your body was addicted to the sugar, fat, and chemicals in processed junk food. Food manufacturers deliberately put high amounts of sugar and flavor additives in their foods so that you will want to buy them and eat them over and over again.

When you stop eating processed foods and start to eat raw and whole foods you will be amazed at how different the food tastes. Not only will you notice that your tastes have altered, but also some foods may even make you feel ill, as if they are literally poisoning you.

People have reported headaches from a reinstatement of unhealthy food into their diets.

Ending the Addiction

Just like a drug addict needs to go through detox to get the drugs out of their system someone who chronically overeats must go through a detox to get that addictive food out of their system.

Once the addictive substances are gone, you are free. You can start to eat the healthy diet you know you should be eating. When that happens, you will be on the path to being truly healthy. You will be able to easily lose weight, and maintain the healthy weight once you have achieved it.

Exercising will become more like fun than work because you will have more energy, and when you are lighter, exercise is less stressful to the body. If you feel yourself starting to return to your former bad habits, you can always go back and do another 3-day detox.

Eating Smaller Portions

You have heard that eating smaller portions is the key to lasting weight loss. After the detox is over you will find that you don't want to eat as much as you did before.

Indeed, you may be physically unable to do so, since during the 3-day liquid diet your stomach will shrink back to normal and you won't need to fill it with so much food to feel full.

The full feeling you may have been used to is an indicator of overindulgence. Did you know that a normal stomach is only about as big as your closed fist?

Think about how much food you eat at every meal. If you are eating much more food at a sitting than the size of a closed fist, you are stretching out your stomach.

You do not need as much food as you think. If you eat slowly, you will notice that your hunger abates before you are so full you have a hard time moving.

Think about how you felt on the last day of your detox. You should now be able to tell the difference between genuine hunger and the myriad of other reasons that you might eat.

An unrealistic estimation of portion size is one of the major reasons why people are so overweight in modern times.

Restaurants routinely provide portions that are 2 to 3 times larger than what a regular portion should be, because people like to feel that they are getting more for their money.

Humans instinctively eat whatever food is available, which once was important for survival, but now is actually detrimental to health.

Restaurants take advantage of this instinct to profit from your ill health. When going out, keep the size of your closed fist in mind as a reference. Ask for a to go box immediately when you sit down, and put all but one reasonable portion in it.

Processed foods also usually have portions that are far too large for the average person. This is probably due to the fact that their nutrition is lacking and they are full of empty calories.

So, you eat much more of them than you should, hoping to get what you need. This is a little like putting cheap gas in your car when you need Premium.

Learning to control your portion size will be a big help in keeping that extra weight off and losing more weight.

When you have finished the 3-day detox you can start eating the kind of diet nutritionists recommend that people should eat for optimum health.

Start eating six small meals a day instead of 3 large meals. Those small meals will fill up your stomach and you won't feel hungry. Your body needs fuel to run, and eating more often means that it will be burning calories for more of the time.

Clean Eating

When your taste for junk food and processed food is gone, you will rediscover the joy of eating real food. Fresh fruits and vegetables, high quality meats, or other protein sources like nuts and soy, will provide you with the nutrition you need to keep you healthy and fit.

Adapting to eating better quality food may require some rearranging of your priorities, but you don't need to make a radical lifestyle change. You don't have to go from eating fast food 3 times a week to growing your own tomatoes and raising your own chickens all in a week.

However, by making small changes in the way that you eat you can take all the lessons you learned from the 3-day detox and use them to transform your life. The 3-day detox can be the start of a truly happy and healthy life for you, no matter how much weight you have to lose.

What to Eat When the Detox is Over

After the detox is done, you will probably be very happy to return to solid food, but don't overdo it. If you run out and get a double cheeseburger, and eat it as fast as you can you will probably make yourself pretty sick.

Eating lots of high calorie, high fat and processed food is what you got into trouble in the first place. So when the detox is done make a commitment to eat better and not stress your body out eating unhealthy food.

When you eat a lot of junk food, it is not just weight gain you have to worry about. Your liver, which breaks down fats and gets rid of toxins for the entire body, can start to break down over time.

Eating a lot of high fat and junk foods can wear out your liver if you're not careful. This is exactly why you chose to do the 3-day detox in the first place.

Eating light and healthy foods will keep your liver working the way it's supposed to and help you stay at a healthy weight.

When the detox is done, you should practice light eating for the next week or so. That way you can maintain the weight loss that you had on the detox and get a good start on a healthier diet.

Light Eating

Light eating means sticking with foods that are healthy and not full of fat or excessive calories. Smaller portions of lighter foods are best for your system after a detox.

You can even add some of the drinks from the detox to your diet in place of meals if you want. Broth and soup are also great light foods to eat, especially if you make them yourself.

For example, if you normally don't have time to eat breakfast you can make up a batch of the breakfast drink from the detox and grab a bottle of that on your way out the door. You will get a healthy breakfast that won't weigh you down. Smoothies are great for quick breakfasts. So are meal replacement bars.

What Foods Are Light Foods?

There are lots of healthy foods that you can add to your diet that are also light. Avoid diet foods that are full of chemicals and artificial sweeteners.

Remember what you learned about cravings? Foods filled with chemicals lead to cravings, because your body isn't getting what it needs. Cravings lead to cheating, and weight gain.

Stick with natural foods that will continue to give your body the energy you had after the detox.

Here is a list of some of the best foods to eat after the detox:

- Raw salads with no dressing or vinaigrette dressing
- Fresh or frozen vegetables
- Fresh fruit
- Whole oats
- Flax seeds
- Vegetable broth
- Soups that are not cream based
- Green Tea
- Protein bars
- Nuts and seeds
- Whole grain crackers

- Organic white meats like chicken or turkey
- Seafood, broiled or grilled
- Nut butters like peanut butter, almond butter, or cashew butter
- Whole grain bread
- Smoothies
- Protein drinks

Light eating without a plan may be difficult for certain people. Just as you did when preparing for the 3-day detox, you may want to have a diet plan in mind for learning about or returning to healthy eating. Without a plan, you may wind up reverting to old habits and gaining back the weight.

So, here is a review of some eating plans you might consider to help you learn to eat the way you should. You'll notice an emphasis among many of them on a total lifestyle change. Isn't that what you wanted to kick start when you began the 3-day detox?

The Atkins Diet

This diet was developed by a doctor, and has science behind it. It proposes that carbohydrates, rather than fat cause weight gain. It focuses on protein, which is proven to help build muscle, which in turn helps burn fat more efficiently.

There are 4 "Phases" to this plan, and a certain amount of carbohydrates allowed at each phase.

The plan uses the restriction of carbohydrates to even out blood sugar spikes and help the body burn calories. The plan has been refined to eliminate unhealthy fats, and includes a maintenance stage that can be an eating plan for life. The down side of this plan is that it is fairly restrictive and may be hard to stick to in the long run.

Cheating really sets you back in this plan. However, if the idea of a long-term plan appeals to you, it is worth checking out in more detail.

The Best Life Diet

Another long-term plan, this one incorporates all elements of your life to assist you making a permanent lifestyle change. It has three phases, and the last is another long-term maintenance plan. This plan requires a serious commitment, as it includes an exercise plan, and a focus on portion control.

On the positive side—the diet is not extremely restrictive. It has a lot of food and exercise options, a generous calorie count, and allows you to tailor it for your needs.

The down side of this plan is that it is not a quick fix (which is honestly how it should be). If a comprehensive plan is for you, look into the Best Life Diet.

The Blood Type Diet

This plan is based upon the idea that each blood type processes food differently. It assumes that if you eat and exercise according to your blood type, you will maintain a healthy weight.

There is much anecdotal evidence for this approach working. However, there is not much science to back it up, beyond what the creator has researched. It could benefit from some independent study.

The Caveman, or Paleo Diet

This one certainly has a buzz around it. The goal of the diet is to train your body to crave healthy foods. It has three stages, one of which is similar to the detox you have already completed! The diet focuses on getting in touch with your body and learning to eat naturally, with whole unprocessed foods.

This one is not about denying yourself and being hungry. It is about eating, but doing it healthily.

The positive? The emphasis on whole foods.

The negative? Entire food groups are left out, so there is a chance of this diet becoming unbalanced.

The French Women Don't Get Fat Diet

This amusingly named plan goes on the supposition that a traditional "diet" with massive restrictions is not necessary. The key to this plan is portion control. It emphasizes examining the quantity of food you eat which should be reduced, and raising the quality of what you consume.

It suggests slowing down and savoring your food, rather than rushing through meals and not even realizing that you are full. There is also an emphasis on hydration, which you have already learned is important. The creator encourages walking everywhere as the only form of exercise required.

The positive elements of this plan are easy to see. You enjoy what you eat. The only foods eliminated are processed foods, and you've already learned that fresh unprocessed food is what your body needs and craves.

The only negatives to this diet are that slowing down is not always an option, and that typically modern life does not allow for the amount of walking prescribed, and that extra exercise may be required.

Glycemic Index Diets

The glycemic index is a scientific ranking of foods comparing how quickly they raise the blood sugar.

Developed for the use of diabetics in controlling their sugar, the glycemic index has influenced mainstream dieting, and spawned several eating plans.

The premise is that foods that raise blood sugar cause fat storage and hunger. Sugar is a High GI food, and all other foods are compared with it when assigning them a value on the Index.

Low GI foods are the healthiest according to this measure, and you should avoid foods with a GI score over 70. However, some food scientists feel that the GI score of the entire meal should be consider rather than each food.

The plan is flexible and has many options, but due to the disagreement over scores, may be difficult to follow.

The Macrobiotic Diet

This is a primarily vegetarian diet, with some seafood allowed. This diet emphasizes fresh foods and locally grown foods, which you already know are preferable.

However, macrobiotic diets are highly restrictive, disallowing red meat, dairy, coffee and several fruits and vegetables. There are tremendous health benefits, but the food is not particularly exciting. You would have to be extremely committed to weight loss and health.

The Mediterranean Diet

Based upon the simple diets observed around the Mediterranean Sea in Greece and Italy, this eating plan emphasizes natural foods, including fresh fruit every day and olive oil as the main source of fat.

It allows lean meat, eggs and dairy. You can even have a glass of red wine! This diet continues to be studied, and compares to low carbohydrate diets in weight loss success. It outperforms low fat diets.

It has many health benefits, lowering your risk of Parkinson's Disease, Alzheimer's, heart disease, cancer and even obesity. The only drawback is the lack of rules.

No food is completely off limits, but some should be moderated. The real trick is learning healthy food preparation. This plan may not provide enough structure for some dieters.

The New Beverly Hill Diet

This eating plan is based on the idea that food doesn't cause people to be overweight. Instead, food inefficiently digested is the culprit. The program relies on eating the right foods at the right time, in the correct combinations. It allows all of the food groups.

However, the rules are fairly complicated, and the combination eating plan is not one that can be maintained. There is also no proof that the plan will work in the long run.

The Shangri-La Diet

The premise of this plan is that you have learned to associate good taste with the calories your body needs for fuel. So you take 1 to 3 tablespoons of olive oil, or 1 to 2 tablespoons of sugar water between meals. You are supposed to eat bland food as well. There are no portion controls. This is supposed to make your body re-learn to eat for nutrition, not taste.

Supposedly you reset your body and learn to be happy with less food. Since no one wants to eat bland foods for an extended period of time, you are very unlikely to be able to stick to the Shangri-La diet long enough for it to work, and it certainly is not a lifestyle that is lasting.

The South Beach Diet

The South Beach Diet was invented by a cardiologist to help his patients lower their risk of heart disease.

At the time, low fat was the diet craze. His research discovered the issue that we have already discussed, that the body needs and craves fat to feel satisfied.

If fat is lacking, the body will demand that you satisfy it by over eating.

The South Beach Diet was designed to be an easy to follow solution for that issue. You simply replace "bad fat", or saturated fat, with "good fat", like unsaturated fat, and our old friend Omega 3.

Additionally, "bad carbs", like processed grains and refined sugar, are replaced with "good carbs", like whole grains and beans. The eating plan has 3 phases, the first phase rather strict, the second phase adding in more of those "good carbs" and the third for maintenance.

The South Beach Diet is intended to be a lifestyle change. The positives? You will not be hungry. Snacking is encouraged, with the idea that over eating comes from getting extremely hungry. The negatives?

As with the Mediterranean Diet, the South Beach Diet very ease and lack of structure is difficult for some dieters who need more structure.

The Volumetrics Diet

A "common sense" eating plan, the Volumetrics Diet looks at the energy density of foods, which is the number of calories in a specific amount. The idea is that if you eat low calorie, high volume food you will feel full.

No foods are off limits, but there is a set number of calories you can eat a day. You are encouraged to do 30 to 60 minutes of exercise per day, and to eat a varied diet. You also should keep a journal. The only possible negative is that it is time consuming to figure out the energy density of your food, and to journal about what you eat.

The Zone Diet

This eating plan is science based, built around a similar idea to the Glycemic Index. The Zone Diet says that food affects hormones which in turn changes insulin production.

The plan maintains that a balance of foods, 40% carbohydrates, 30% protein, and 30% fat will place your body into the Zone, the metabolic state that is efficient.

Although there are suggested calorie limits, the focus is on maintaining the ratios. 30 minutes of exercise, 6 days a week is a part of the Zone lifestyle.

Despite accusations of junk science, there is massive anecdotal evidence that The Zone Diet works. There are no significant negatives reported.

Although this appears to be a great deal of information, upon reading through the plans you will see that the ones that work are those based on the same principles we have been talking about, reducing your caloric intake and raising your rate of exercise.

The plans listed have varying amounts of structure depending on what you need. So, when you are ready to move from light eating to the healthy lifestyle you wish to maintain, you will be armed with the information to help you.

Exercising After the 3-day Detox

As we've been discussing, if you want to keep up your weight loss after the detox, you should start adding more exercise to your day. You don't need to start spending hours in the gym, or train for a marathon.

However, you will find that you have more energy after the detox. Don't waste it! You can put some of that energy into getting fit.

Getting fit has many benefits for your continued health, aside from the fact that it will help you continue to lose weight and look more toned. Fitness speeds up your metabolism, which you have already cranked up with the 3-day detox!

Being fit gives you energy, and can help prevent heart disease and stroke. It can help you manage arthritis pain. Fitness is an excellent hedge against depression, as regular physical activity elevates your mood naturally.

Regular exercise can help you sleep, as long as you don't do it too close to bed time. When you combine exercise with lighter eating in your new lifestyle, you will find it easy to keep up a healthy weight.

Although most authorities advise 30 minutes of physical activity per day, to start out getting more exercise you can use activities that you already like to do.

Make time to get out and spend some quality time with your family and friends doing things like:

- Hiking
- Swimming
- Walking
- Playing sports
- Dancing
- Riding bikes
- Joining a gym
- Going to yoga classes

Exercise certainly can and should be something that you can enjoy and not dread. After the detox you will have a lot more energy and your joints and muscles won't ache as badly as they did.

If none of these choices appeals to you, get creative with your cardio. Find a workout video you like, or simply watch your favorite show while you walk on the treadmill!

There are simple circuit workouts that you can do from home with minimal equipment. Remember that as long as each session lasts at least 10 minutes, cardio training is cumulative throughout the day. Many public pools have water aerobics classes.

As long as you are moving, you will gain some benefit. Even house work, like scrubbing floor and changing sheets, or yard work, like raking and weeding, burn calories and add to your fitness level.

The more you exercise after doing the detox the more you will enjoy exercise. Success breeds success, just like you discovered during your time spent detoxing.

Finally, you can have the healthy and active lifestyle that you always wanted. And all it starts with the 3-day detox!

Chapter Eight

Do It Again

Did you know you can do the 3-day detox more than once? You can. You can do it again to prepare for another event. You can also do it again on a regular basis to clean out your body and maintain your weight and your health.

Many people find that they feel so good after the 3-day detox they want to do it again to stay healthy.

Nutritionists recommend a detox every few months to help your body clean itself out, but most people do not bother because they think detoxes are difficult. You know better.

You shouldn't do the detox two weekends in a row because it is hard on the body.

Some experts advise only doing a serious detox 2 or 3 times a year, some say once every 3 months is safe.

Listen to your body. If you have recovered from your last 3-day detox, and then begin feeling sluggish and out of sorts as you did before, then it might be time to repeat the process.

I hope you have learned something from this book so far and would greatly appreciate it if you could leave an honest review on Amazon.com.

Discover Scientifically-Proven "Shortcuts" & "Hacks" to Lose Weight FASTER (With Very Little Effort)

For this month only, you can get Linda's best-selling & most popular book absolutely free – *Weight Loss Secrets You NEED to Know*.

Get Your FREE Copy Here:
TopFitnessAdvice.com/Bonus

Discover scientifically-proven tips to help you lose weight faster and easier than ever before. With this book, readers were able to improve their weight loss results and fitness levels. So, it's highly recommended that you get this book, especially while it's free!

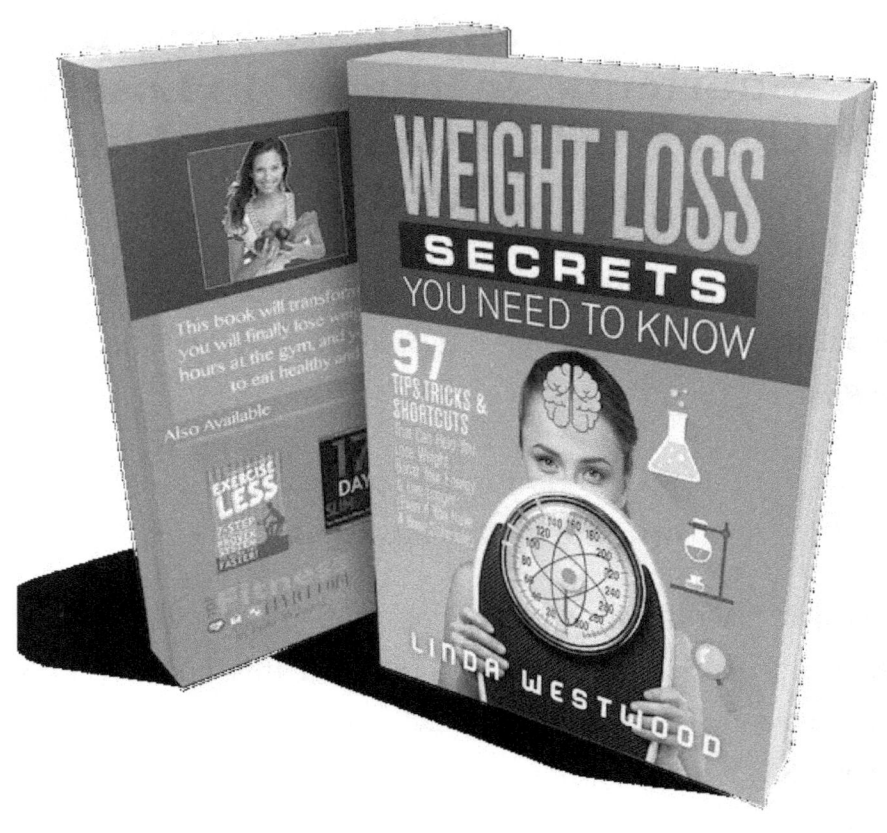

Get Your FREE Copy Here:

TopFitnessAdvice.com/Bonus

Conclusion

The 3-day detox is a challenge, yet it is an effective method to combat some of the biggest obstacles you face when trying to lose weight.

In review, these conditions will put up a roadblock in front of your weight loss. The 3-day detox does the job of a demolition crew, knocking these obstructions out your way and clearing your body to lose the weight you want to lose.

The detox can clear up body pollution, which are those toxins, impurities and other unhealthy leftovers your body can hold on to from years of overeating, a poor, junk food diet, and little exercise.

Body pollution can completely stall your weight loss, because your body's waste elimination systems are clogged, sluggish and unable to function.

The 3-day detox powerfully flushes all of the pollutants out of your system.

The 3-day detox combats a slow metabolism, which may result from your health habits or your age, using ingredients that crank up your metabolism, such as green tea, blueberries, spinach and kale.

These superfoods will get your motor running in high gear and head you straight toward the healthy lifestyle change you need to lose weight and feel great!

Best of all, the 3-day detox can help kick start your weight loss. You can lose up to 10 pounds while working on the 3-day detox. That is an entire dress size in just a weekend.

You will look and feel great for your event, or just for you! What better way is there to begin your transformation to a slimmer healthier you?

Final Words

I would like to thank you for purchasing my book and I hope I have been able to help you and educate you on something new.

If you have enjoyed this book and would like to share your positive thoughts, could you please take 30 seconds of your time to go back and give me a review on my Amazon book page.

I greatly appreciate seeing these reviews because it helps me share my hard work.

You can leave me a review on Amazon.com.

Again, thank you and I wish you all the best!

Enjoying this book?

Check out my other best sellers!

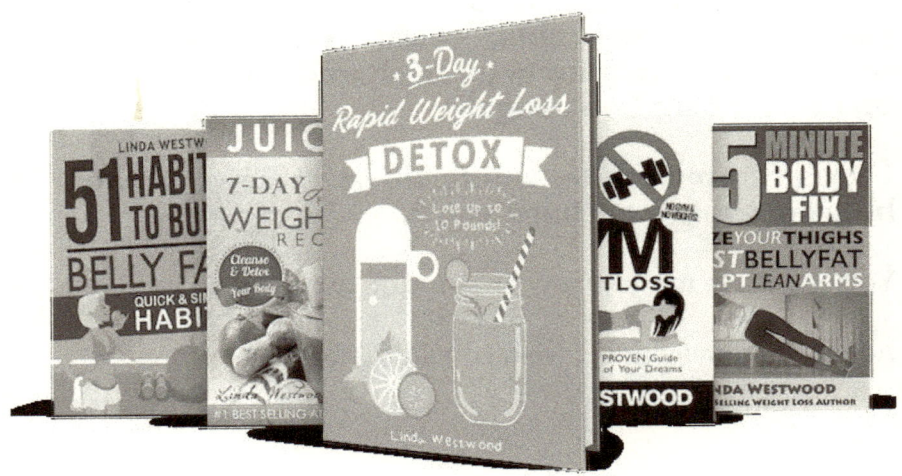

Get your next book on sale here:

TopFitnessAdvice.com/go/books

www.ingramcontent.com/pod-product-compliance
Lightning Source LLC
Chambersburg PA
CBHW031155020426
42333CB00013B/684